Coping with Research   JAN. 1988

Other books by James Calnan:

One Way to do Research
Speaking at Medical Meetings
Writing Medical Papers
How to Speak and Write
Talking With Patients

COPING WITH RESEARCH

The complete guide for beginners

James Calnan
FRCS, FRCP

Emeritus Professor of Plastic and Reconstructive Surgery
University of London
at the
Royal Postgraduate Medical School
and
Hammersmith Hospital, London

William Heinemann Medical Books
London

DISCLAIMER

Without disrespect, I have used the male pronoun throughout. I realise that my writing is for both sexes, but to indicate this continually in English is clumsy.

ISBN 0–433–05014–4

First published in Great Britain in 1984 by
William Heinemann Medical Books Ltd,
23 Bedford Square,
London WC1B 3HH

Typeset by Inforum Ltd, Portsmouth
and printed in Great Britain by
Redwood Burn Ltd, Trowbridge, Wilts.

CONTENTS

Chapter 9.   A THESIS

Chapter 10.   THE SUMMING UP

PREFACE

I have waited 25 years for this book to be written, by someone else. I needed it, to give to the many who asked advice on how to start research. Doctors, nurses, physiotherapists, speech therapists, psychologists, educationalists, teachers, trainers and pupils all want to do their own thing. And why not? The young and keen have good ideas but need a little help to get started. Some need help to continue.

It is commonly said that good research cannot be taught. It is also said that most people would like to do research but do not have the time for it. So where does good research come from? From those who make time and take the trouble to learn how. In spite of all the difficulties, the amount of successful research as judged by publications – and research without publication is sterile – is increasing all the time. For medicine the amount doubles in about seven years!

This book tries to make your research planning, performance and publication easier. It will not do the work for you, but may help you to get started and well-organised. More than anything, I hope that it will give you a feeling for style in all that you do: a style that will be yours, a style that others will appreciate, a feeling for excellence that is immediately obvious because you enjoy style. And may you keep your sense of fun and let a little appear in your thinking, speaking and writing. This book is for beginners only.

JAMES CALNAN

1

TO GET YOU STARTED

One of the good things about the world in which we live is the amount of encouragement we receive to "do it yourself". The mysteries of a host of different jobs, cooking and car maintenance, dressmaking and plumbing, growing your own vegetables and assembling your own furniture are all opened up to ordinary people like you and me by means of the magic instruction manual. These come in two forms: the very simple and the extremely complicated. But they all claim to enable us to master the job in hand. If we do all that the instruction manual tells us to – no more and no less – we should end up with a product we can be proud of. Indeed, we can become experts just by following the instructions; if we persevere for long enough we become masters. Instant expertise has been so publicised that many people expect too much: "add water and stir" is all that some expect to do to produce cuisine that others have spent a lifetime trying to perfect.

Why devote a book to beginners? Apart from the obvious, that we all have to begin somewhere – and a book is as good a place as any, and better than most casual advice – there are two reasons. First, beginners have the chance to pick up good habits and develop a healthy scepticism, whereas those established in research have learnt to cut corners and enjoy it and are therefore unteachable in many ways; beginners start with a clean canvas upon which they may sketch the outline of what they want to do and how they want to do it. Second, within the concept of a general craft there are of course many specialist crafts included in the spectrum of research, such as medical, nursing, managerial and so on. There is need of a simple and practical book for the beginner which will not only set him on the right road but give him an idea of style, of elitism, of self-confidence, of precision in thinking, of appreciation of the geniuses who brought us so far to the present age of technology. Although this book is biased towards medical research, the general principles are applicable just as effectively to the accountant, architect, industrialist and many others. Understand that medicine is not a science, it is a technology and a pretty successful one at that, but only because it has developed and used the right tools. Medicine in the eighteenth century was much the same as that in ancient Rome – twentieth-century medicine is vastly different.

Hence a book can guide you and set you in the right direction. Doing research is practising the art, because we all learn better by doing and not just by reading or watching others. Sooner rather than later you will need a personal guide, a teacher, adviser, mentor, spiritual director – call him or her what you will – someone who has travelled further and more widely in your chosen subject, and who can offer encouragement to advance. Some will say: "I would like to do research but I've no idea how to start". How strong is the desire? This book may help. Others will say: "I would like to do research but cannot find the time". The kindest advice is to say don't bother: but what does he do with his time and his mind? You'll be amazed how much of the day is spent doing nothing. This is not boredom! Boredom is not doing nothing, but having nothing to do. The former is occasionally compulsory and profitable, the latter never.

WHY DO RESEARCH?

Why do research? You won't get paid for writing an important article on your findings, indeed you may have the greatest difficulty in getting it published. The reward for long hours and disappointment, for working on a project when others are playing or relaxing, is not money: it is achievement. If you don't enjoy it, why do it? In research you have joined an exclusive club of people who ask questions and then go on to find answers.

Sir Kenneth Dover[17] wrote about the Greeks of two thousand years ago: "They were resilient, sceptical, cheeky people, whose distinctive contribution to our history was to combine a readiness to ask 'Why?' and 'Why not?', with a conviction that only some reasoned and clearly expounded answers to those questions were worth listening to". Researchers follow the same philosophy: good questions and good answers. We should continually question traditional practices and take nothing for granted, as we will discuss in the next chapter. But in the end, research is an act of faith,[2,3,7,8,10] the faith that we live in an organised world, the world is rational, there is such a thing as cause and effect, but the cause comes before the effect, that knowledge can be discovered and can be added to, that problems are soluble, and truth is real but absolute truth is unattainable: there is no foreseeable end. The belief that experiment is a practical and productive procedure, that research can bring benefits to us and to our fellows, that research is intellectual nourishment because it contains the challenge, "why?", and finally that research is fun. You can argue that there is no good evidence for any of these articles of faith, but you will argue in vain. Researchers know.

CAN RESEARCH BE TAUGHT?

Professional researchers encounter one misconception more often than any other: that their art is something that cannot be taught. But all art is achieved through the exercise of a craft, and every craft has rudiments that must be taught. The craft of research is no exception. The problem is trying to find a way to teach efficiently and effectively. Moreover, the effort of teaching must be seen to be worthwhile, both by the teacher and by the taught. The talent is there but untapped because conventional methods of teaching research are unsatisfactory and, unless they are adapted by some exceptional teacher, fail to give students any guidance in the art of passing on their own newly-acquired knowledge. One must have a real idea of what makes creative research live, of how advances are made and why research is important. The same arguments apply to fine-art painting, yet one way by which some skills are readily acquired is by the technique called "painting by numbers".

Many people are interested in fine art and would enjoy painting in oils, but cannot draw. Books tell them that it is not necessary to be able to draw, that the painting will take shape as they observe and apply colours. This is hard to believe and there are many who have tried and found what they expected, a mess. To overcome this difficulty – and everyone can recognise bad drawing, incorrect perspective, and dull composition at a glance – painting by numbers was invented. Frowned on by the 'experts', condemned as non-creative, it became an immediate success.

You can buy a canvas, mounted and primed, in which there is drawn (for example) a bowl of spring flowers set on a mahogany table against the background of a draped velvet curtain: a classical still-life. Each flower is not only drawn well but the various parts of the bloom are sketched in and numbered. Hence, one petal or one leaf will have several subdivisions each with its own number. The job of the "artist" is to mix the correct colour and apply within the designated area. The same colour is required in several different places and as a result the disparate application of one colour establishes a sense of unity as the picture is built up. The painter has a choice in the way he applies his paint: it can be put on thin or thick, confined entirely within the drawn area or allowed to overlap the next.

There is a sense of discovery and of adventure. Leonardo da Vinci is said to have smudged his oil painting and accidentally discovered aerial perspective: that things far away are less sharp than those nearer, not out of focus but with blurred edges, and if outdoors they appear bluer than things nearer.

What has all this to do with research? Quite a lot. But consider the number of things the artist, painting by numbers, is likely to obtain.

First, he has acquired a tangible piece of art, the result of his own diligence and ability, which he can varnish, frame and hang on his wall. There will be natural pride in accomplishment. He did it and so can you. The artist knows, instinctively, that he can do it again and probably better: if the picture gives pleasure to his friends he certainly will repeat the oil painting, and each will be different. He has gained confidence and the interest and encouragement to do better next time, the resolve to continue the new found skills.

Second, he has acquired knowledge of the technique of applying oil paint. Walter Gropius said: "so much for techniques what about beauty?". Well, beauty is style; beauty is a personal thing and so is style. You can recognise both when you see them, but they are easier to recognise if you have tried to create them yourself, and discovered that there is more to oil painting than meets the eye and therefore a stimulus to look deeper. But in painting flowers you begin to learn more about them: their shapes, textures, colours, individualities, postures, their names, and so develop an interest in botany which was never intentional. There is no such thing as right and wrong in the absolute sense, but you can tell the difference in your own work even though it may be difficult to explain to another.

Third, the painter learns a lot about colours: their moods, imagery, tone, freshness, hue, harmony and infinite variety. Some colours appear to recede, others to advance towards the viewer. They can be blended to produce new magic, or mud, but care in application, taking one step at a time, not rushing, becomes an obvious necessity for success even though it is mainly self-discipline imposed from within oneself; and there develops a feeling for composition and harmony which would be difficult to learn from another because these are abstract ideas.

Fourth, painting a picture will make you see things you never saw before, things you would not have seen if you had not been painting, either because you never looked for them or because nobody had pointed them out.

Finally, a sense of creation. The artist started with paint, brushes and canvas but ended with an oil painting, something that he created. There is also a little of the meaning of art in the act of creation. Admittedly fine art is a knack rather than a skill, at least in part; some of it clearly can't be taught. No one can really explain what it is you do to produce a picture which has a certain quality that makes it stand out from others. One moment you can't do it, it's impossible; then suddenly you did it, can do it, and can't explain how. And once you've learnt you don't forget. But you need to learn the basics in order to produce something creative and tangible, yet good art cannot be taught because knack and flair are required. It is not enough to sit and think, although that comes into it too. Moreover, an oil painting can communicate to a viewer in various ways: at technical, spiritual, emotional and allegorical levels – the artist puts these on his canvas too, even if they are not immediately obvious.

So the painter has learnt five things which he did not know before. All of them have parallels for the researcher because, in practice, research and painting are both adventures of exploration. Don Quixote once asked a painter what he was painting. "That", he replied, "is as may turn out to be". For painting that says it all, for research it is not enough because we have to know what to expect. Art, says the dictionary, is skill as a result of knowledge and practice. Whenever one makes or does something with skill and with concern for its excellence, one becomes an artist. The craft of research is an art form which must be practised regularly, yet research is also an adventure like a painting for if we knew beforehand precisely how it would turn out we would in all likelihood never begin.

Many people are interested in research but do not know how to begin. Although it is not possible to provide an outline drawing and a book of instructions with a photograph of the finished product as we can for the artist, it is possible to outline the technical stages and indicate where help may be obtained. Unlike the diffident artist who needs the draughted composition on which to apply his colours, the beginner in research has the "bare bones" of an idea but cannot supply the muscles, skin and clothes to make it come alive.[3,10,40] So we come back to the original question, can research be taught? This book is an expression of the faith that it can, or at least the basics. One of the oldest questions in research institutes is whether research skills are self-taught or learnt from others. But there are several skills involved. The "Do it Yourself" fashion cannot be applied to creation of ideas but can to much else, even though there is no instruction manual which guarantees success. So, what do we mean by research?

WHAT IS RESEARCH?

Research is "an investigation directed to the discovery of some fact by careful study of a subject", and it can mean "a course of critical or scientific inquiry". Hence a researcher is an investigator, a detective. That is the general dictionary definition. But there are other definitions which are more helpful because they give an insight into the spirit or ethos behind what is often called scientific research. A medical dictionary calls research "scientific investigation, the establishment of facts and their significance by experiment, and the scientific collection of and analysis of data". But when we look up "science" in the same dictionary we find the term defined as a body of accepted fact; "any system of knowledge covering a special field of investigation", because it comes from the Latin word *scientia*, meaning knowledge.

The fundamentals of research can be stated in one sentence. Research is the making of observations, proposing an hypothesis to explain them, testing the hypothesis by experiment, and reaching a conclusion. It is the practical application of scientific method, often more but never less. Of course there are difficulties. The observations may be incorrect, inaccurate or incomplete; the hypothesis may be formulated wrongly, the tests impossible and the conclusions not understandable.

Yet this way of research has very wide application – for medicine, for industry, for science itself, for everyday life. It is the way of progress. In research there is a well-tried step-by-step way of doing things and of thinking; the details may change but not the sequence. Indeed there is a common thread running through the weave of a simple comparative trial of a new form of management and the most complicated, expensive, multidisciplinary investigation of a life-saving drug: all statements must be substantiated by evidence.

The recipe for successful research on the other hand, is delightfully simple: hard work and a bloody good idea. In the end, successful research is being the first to state the obvious. However, it is technology rather than science, which teaches us to retain the things that work and discard the things that don't. The primary canon in research, as in education, is to arouse interest; indeed the value of research to most people lies in education and to get research off the ground you will need four things:-

1. Some useful personal qualities, such as curiosity, enthusiasm, and talent.
2. An original idea.
3. Access to a specialist library.
4. A person to talk to, someone to help you get started, a mentor.

If you have none of these, stop reading: research is not for you.

Opportunity and luck count for much but, without these four, research can be very difficult. When to start? Now. Age is a most unreliable method of measuring capabilities. J.R.R. Tolkien wrote that "it's the job that never started that takes the longest to finish", and this is all too true of research. If there is an idea niggling in your mind, looking for an answer then you may need a push to get started but the real question should be how to start?

THE PERSONAL VALUE OF RESEARCH

Although this book is about how to get started and how to do research, it is worth spending a little time to consider the benefits of doing research or at least of being exposed to research. Research will give you a wider horizon in your job, one which you could not have acquired in any other way, and it does give you a view of science which can be exciting in itself. The discipline of research which requires you to take a single thought, examine it in depth and read the necessary literature will improve personal technique and performance in whatever job you have. As Bernard Leach, a famous potter in his time, used to say: "Whatever a man does well makes a better man".

There are also several practical rewards. By learning to use statistics intelligently one's judgement improves; the nature of an experiment will develop imagination and a comparative trial between two methods of management –

a word used in its widest sense – may help to change or confirm your attitudes. I am aware of the expression that "attitudes resist change, that is their function", but attitudes should be based on supported fact and not on religious faith. Perhaps the most important reward is that you can acquire three skills that every educated person should have: the ability to read critically, how to speak well, and how to write comprehensible English. These then are the "spin offs" from personal research.

A MENTOR

Successful research depends on two things above all: a library from which to seek others' mistakes and knowledge, and a wealth of experience in your own subject. But the beginner, almost by definition, lacks experience, so how will he compensate? By having a mentor and making full use of him. That is by choosing someone who will supply the missing knowledge, information, direction, and experience; so someone rather special like the "preceptor" in the last century – the sponsor and usually a family doctor – required by every medical student, whom the student would seek to emulate and to whom he could turn throughout his studies.

Is it possible to teach yourself successful research? Can you become your own tutor? Yes. But you will find life that much harder and lonelier. Not everything can be learnt because successful research will depend on experience, judgement and diligence. The novice may have plenty of the third but will lack the other two. This is where the mentor comes in: he provides enough of the missing ingredients to guarantee momentum. Bismarck's advice should be heeded: "Only a fool learns from experience, the trick is to learn from the experience of others." Even so, experience without talent is useless for, as Aldous Huxley wrote, "Experience is not what happens to you: it is what you do with what happens to you."

Take care in the choice of your mentor. He may be the most important choice of your life and decide the quantity, quality, and style of your future work, so take your time. Decide what you need in the way of support and make discreet inquiries. He must have a good "track record" of personal research and publications, and of helping others with both of these. Four special qualities are particularly important.

First, a confidant to whom you can talk freely in the sure knowledge that what you say is strictly confidential. You are bound to need someone who is interested in you and your future, who believes in you; invariably a warm relationship develops, so it has to be someone whom you can get on with for you may have to bare your soul. You must feel at ease with your mentor, have confidence in him, enjoy his company and come away refreshed and excited from any discussion. Hero-worship is not a bad thing; a good mentor will take pride in your achievements by telling you and other people about your successes.

You need someone to check your ideas and make you explain them in such detail that you define and refine them until you reach clarity of thought. As Charles Causeley wrote, someone to sort out:-

"The trendy and the mad,
The feeble and the downright bad."

The mentor will help throughout your research, but at the ideas stage he will be of special value because you may be able with assistance to expand your own ideas and go further than expected – he will be a teacher of the spirit and style of research, someone who understands your subject and so can monitor your performance, give advice on how to proceed and thus help with planning. He will tell you who to go and see, who to talk to, and then provide the necessary introductions.

Second, someone who gives advice when asked, but you

must ask because you alone can decide whether to accept. He may see your problem with different eyes and offer a solution you had not thought of. He will also help you write you paper, prepare your lecture, compose your grant application – if you ask. He will supply the missing experience and provide value-judgements; he will criticise but offer constructive criticism, comfort you when things go wrong, and encourage you to continue when all looks black.

Third, someone who will make time to see you and give of his time sufficient for your needs at that moment. He will often be busy himself, indeed he may be the busiest and most productive man on site, yet manages to find ample time to listen to you and give advice. Never discuss half-baked ideas, half-drawn plans, first drafts of papers or lectures: you waste a valuable resource, his time.

Fourth, look for two special qualities in your mentor: vision and awareness. A man with a vision of the future, of the possibilities of your own project, will infect you with his own enthusiasm. The mentor who is aware of work in a similar field to that of your own can save you much time, but it is someone with a general feeling of awareness of what is happening in the world outside your institution that you need most. Insularity is mental, physical and emotional. And bad.

But however much you take advice, in the end you must make the decision whether to accept or reject that advice. You have to carry out the research – it cannot be done by proxy – and so only you can decide how you will do it. Never ask advice unless you intend to take it. You needn't use it, because you are not a puppet to do the bidding of a senior, but you must have the intention: without that there can be no judgement.

Know this: a teacher's help is desirable, but you *can* tackle research on your own. It is that much harder to start and that much likelier not to be finished. Remember too that good mentors are rare, and very precious. Never knowingly manipulate or deceive yours – you may never get another.

> It is far more difficult to be simple than to be complicated, far more difficult to sacrifice skill and cease exertion in the proper place, than to expend both indiscriminately.
>
> John Ruskin

2

IDEAS

Central to the act of research is the idea, for without an idea there can be no research, or at least no need to do research. If it's knowledge we want then we can look it up in an encyclopaedia, just as the novelist does for details of the country he has never visited. Research requires two things: an idea and the means to test it.

So where do ideas come from? From the top of your head. They are the results of your imagination.[3,10,39,41,63,65] Simple isn't it? Well, not quite because if you look up the meaning of the word "idea" in the dictionary – a good place to start – you will find that it means "conception". Now, conception implies that it was conceived and original, and that implies that it started as an embryo thought. What we want are three processes: first, a means to develop our embryo idea to maturity; second, some simple tests to apply to find whether our infant idea is likely to be any good; and third, a means whereby we can hold up our idea for all the world to see, adopt, or criticise, but with supporting evidence to show that we are right.

Ideas and concepts, we treat both the same, imply originality even though originality is a pretty rare quality. The adage that "there is nothing new under the sun" is to be found in many languages of this world (I know of only four) and there are plenty of people waiting to tell you that it can't be done when you have prepared definite experiments.

Don't worry. It's your idea. Few ideas are original in an absolute sense but many are relatively new and hence the queue of people waiting to patent new inventions. There are some people who cannot think of an idea on their own, but will develop one provided by someone else. The reason is painfully simple: they are less imaginative, or more precisely they lack powers of observation and sensitivity. They may be less clever, or it may be that they have not spent a lifetime with their eyes and ears open and their mental antennae finely tuned to what goes on around them. It takes all sorts to do research, perhaps one of its greatest attractions: addiction is the more appropriate word.

There is an old adage that researchers fall into two categories: ordinary people in extraordinary circumstances (luck?) and extraordinary people in ordinary circumstances (genius?). Some critics would say that research today suffers from too many ordinary people with ordinary ideas in ordinary situations. Do not be put off by these desk-bound critics. There are reluctant researchers, spasmodic researchers and even lapsed researchers, but there is always room for new entrants whatever their temperament.

CREATIVITY

With ideas, we have introduced the concept of creativity, and creativity seems to depend on ten things:

• An ability to see a relationship between bits of knowledge, something which others cannot see, and then to join them up to produce a new idea.

• An ability to alter the environment and then be able to see and study one process only.

• The facility to measure or devise a means of measuring natural phenomena.

• The art of recognising comparisons and realising their possibilities.

• A knack of devising new methods for testing processes or materials.

- An active rejection rather than a passive acceptance of the status quo.

- An attitude which dispels the idea of ambiguity and uncertainty – statistics admits both – a kind of intolerance which insists on resolving this unsatisfying state.

- Some know more than others, have a wider view of the subject and so can see further ahead, and eventually we catch up with them. We call them people "ahead of their time" and when we do catch up we wonder why they were ever thought to be outstanding.

- There are some who have a certain awareness of what goes on around us, perhaps more curiosity in the things we take for granted.

- Finally, there are some who have talent, a knack or perhaps pure luck to hit on the right idea at the right time when such is awaited.

But back to originality because not much research is truly original, yet the majority of research is worthwhile. What is original must be individual; it is different. Originality also means one who encounters the origin of his work within his individual experience of the imagination and the work carries the conviction of authority. For all that, there is now ample evidence that several individuals can hit on the same new idea at the same time, and quite independently. The result is often a clash of personalities for priority of claim.

We all know that a spark can start a bush fire and metaphorically a spark can start an idea in our head. Where does the spark come from? The stimulation of ideas is multifactorial: from personal observation, talking, lectures, discussions, reading, writing about a specific subject or more generally, personal inquisitiveness, and dreaming. The dreamer has a lot to offer when he dreams of the right things because he may see an old problem in a new light and with a new solution. Reverie is not the same as sleep: it is not idle if an original written statement comes out of it.

TYPES OF RESEARCH

Bright ideas come in various forms – large, medium, small, and minute; and in various types – ordinary, stale, promising, and crazy; but the essential question is, can we classify research ideas or at least group them together? Probably not completely, but having outlined the creative process we can note that ideas tend to fall into three categories.

First, there is research that questions current practice. This form has wide application, to professions, trades, and in the home. For instance, there is nothing wrong with the company treasurer asking why certain drugs are used by certain doctors when published research implies or states openly that those drugs are useless. Of course, as soon as this question is posed there will be the cry of "interference with clinical freedom", and we have to admit that freedom often means traditional practice with no incentive to change. We are dealing with attitudes, and attitudes are resistant to change – that is their function.

We can question our own actions and processes: do they do what they are supposed to do? If not, why not? Can practical methods be improved, simplified, made more economical or more exact? As Medawar[40] pointed out, most original research begins with Baconian experimentation to find out more about what we are studying.

Second, there is research that looks for a problem and then proposes a solution. In commerce this is often the quick way to become a millionaire: to discover a need and be the first to satisfy it.

Third, research that produces totally new concepts is the most difficult type of research because it requires an unusual kind of imagination. Imagination cannot work in a vacuum: there must be something to be imaginative about, usually a background of observation. Konrad Lorenz is the living proof that eccentric, inspired guesses are frequently the basis of scientific progress. Although told by his professor of anatomy to continue his studies, he preferred to observe animal behaviour and was awarded the Nobel Prize for Medicine in 1973 (shared with Nikolaas Tinbergen and Karl von Frisch). He did what he enjoyed, what interested him, and founded a whole new discipline of ethology: he was controversial, assertive, flamboyant, and became the world's leading animal watcher.

Yet we should be conscious of Sir Karl Popper's advice[39,50] to a young researcher. It was not, "Go round and observe" in the hope that an original idea would spring to mind. What a good teacher says is this: "Try to learn what people are discussing nowadays in science. Find out where difficulties arise, and take an interest in disagreements. These are the questions which you should take up." In other words, study the problem situation of the day, because we live in a complex world and there is no wisdom to tell us and no scientific tradition to help us choose the right question to ask. All we can do is to see where and how other people started and where they got to. A consequence of always starting from problems, real problems which actually exist and have to be grappled with, is that we become committed to our research. Popper put the greatest premium on boldness of imagination because that allows advances in a jump instead of the amoeba-like movement in the normal evolution of ideas. But big jumps evoke big criticisms.

The Duke of Edinburgh once said that 99% of his new ideas never bore fruit; many would think that with a 1% success rate he is fortunate. All bright ideas have a high mortality so how can we tell if our idea is a good one and likely to provide us with a viable research project? By applying in sequence five simple tests. It is not enough just to have an idea; it has to pass certain preliminary tests before it can be considered seriously.

THE FIVE PRELIMINARY TESTS

●**The writing test**.   We all think in language, sometimes diagrammatic, sometimes numerical but usually in words of our native tongue and that is where there may be trouble. "Noise" in information theory means anything which detracts from or interferes with the passing of information and semantic "noise" concerns language, but it is within your power to deal with that. You will have to encode your idea in language, transmit the IDEA in the right medium to another person, who will decode it and hopefully receive the same idea that you had in your head. If you can write a brief synopsis describing your idea you will have advanced one more step in the right direction. The original IDEA will be modified just a little because it has been transformed from a vague and rather abstract concept to something more concrete written on a piece of paper. After the synopsis, write a suitable title: you now have given a "handle" to your idea. If you can't put it down on paper, the IDEA is probably unreal and not worth pursuing. So the first real test is an order: write it down.

●**The credibility test**. Does it fit in with current knowledge of the subject? Does it make sense? It may be incredible and difficult to accept when it does fit observed fact, so it is important to check the original observations if the new idea was derived from them because observations can easily be false. One of the most difficult things to do in this life is to make an accurate observation.

●**The friendly colleague test**.   Talk to a friend working in the same field, or at least someone who knows your subject, and ask what he thinks. Is it crazy? Does he understand it? Is it good? If you have a mentor discuss it with him. Don't be afraid to discuss ideas and to seek opinions. Many fear that others will steal the IDEA, work on it and deprive them of the claim to originality. Occasionally this does happen, but more than likely you will receive help and encouragement from people who have their own problems to solve and are not anxious to take on more; and they may point out the difficulties. But as René and Jean Dubos have written: "In science, the credit goes to the man who convinces the world, not to the man to whom the idea first occurs". Of course there are people who say "it can't be done" in every walk of life; you are not looking for those, but for a dispassionate appraisal. The IDEA will change a little as you reshape it from the opinion of others.

●**The freshness test**.   Is it new? The only way to find out – and the answer is likely to be "no" – is to conduct a library search. Start with standard textbooks that will tell you whether the subject has been well investigated or is still a problem; they will also provide key reference publications which you should read. Ask the librarian, your mentor and colleagues for leads into the relevant literature; even information about the right journal to thumb through can be a valuable tip. The IDEA may now suffer a very radical alteration. More than likely your reading of the journals has sharpened the IDEA and trimmed it to a more practical proposition.

●**The possibility test**.   Finally, is it possible to do? Can enough instances be studied? Do we have sufficient basic knowledge? Is it falsifiable? Will a statistician have to be consulted about the number of cases that have to be studied before coming to a decision? The answer to this question is "you should" but most people don't. The IDEA may need to be reshaped. More importantly can I do it with my limited knowledge, facilities, help, money? Is it too complex to do alone? Am I the right person to attempt it? The IDEA may need to be modified yet again. Is it important or trivial? Will it lead anywhere, or affect other people? Is there preliminary work to do? The IDEA has now come into proper focus.

So, after each test your original idea has changed, sometimes imperceptibly, sometimes radically. Indeed, you may no longer consider it very original but it is still your idea, your creation. Now you can begin to formulate a plan of how to make the IDEA into a research project and how to test it by experiment. It may be worth embarking on the research in a small way at first, as a pilot trial.

Although the various tests have been given as a list, they can be thought of "in the round" almost all at once as "brain patterns".[9] Take a sheet of paper and write the main idea in the centre. Encircle it. Now draw lines branching from the centre representing an associated idea or test and labelled appropriately. In this way it is possible to keep the main idea under review and show its interconnections.

One of the objectives of all these tests is to avoid working on a second-hand, clapped-out project, and the only way to make sure you don't is to ask the people who can recognise the best: second-best is for others. Few research projects change their shape dramatically as they pass these various tests, but they change enough so that when you look back you can say to yourself: that was a worthwhile improvement, I'm glad I went along with it. The final decision rests with you, it always does, but only a fool will not listen and weigh up advice, whether he accepts it or not.

DUFF GEN

In the wartime, RAF rumours were common: the squadron was moving to another airfield, ops were scrubbed, someone was missing, and so on. All false information and we called it duff gen. Today similar alarms occur in newspapers: epidemics, breakthroughs, revolutionary new methods, and for a while we believe them and are disturbed. The same occurs in research, but in research duff gen is serious. It occupies space in libraries and in men's minds where instead there should be truth. And it provides opportunities for research projects. The project may lead to a negative result and therefore be difficult to get published, but if the techniques whereby the result was obtained has general application, a worthwhile advance has been made.

Where do these false ideas come from? Few are deliberate misinformation, most evolve from errors of interpretation, and some flow from wrong premises.

● False statements are made in the belief that they are true, because making sure of all the facts takes time and trouble.

● There is insufficient evidence and more work is required to reach a firm conclusion, but support for an idea is suggested though not proven by the facts. There is no deliberate deception of others, rather self-deception which others accept.

● There may be suppression of the truth because the temptation to suppress evidence which does not fit in with a preconceived hypothesis is very real. It is easy to select observations and evidence which support one hypothesis, and ignore inconvenient choices.

● The slanting of news and views, by interpreting results and explanation in a certain way, by jumping to conclusions, is common in everyday life.

● Deliberate lies, on the basis that anything is permissible which is successful.

If all this sounds like paranoia then we should remember that each has been well documented in the past ten years. There are any number of cases purporting to prove one thing, taken up by the media and disseminated widely, where refutation becomes extremely difficult to get accepted especially if commercial, industrial or emotional interests are concerned.[19]

If, as frequently happens, the support for an hypothesis is not acceptable, the publication of the results of research and the subsequent criticism of the methods and conclusions should ensure that any wholly or partly false information does not come to be accepted. "But, there is a very serious weakness in this argument because the author of the paper and the critic both have vested interests in the subject. The same factors which may have led the one astray might conceivably have led the other from the narrow path as well and probably the most powerful of the factors is wishful thinking or the desire to make the results of research conform to the postulated theory".[19] Amen to that!

THE DEFINITIVE TEST

The classical concept of scientific method is quite simple and logical. One starts with an observation and tries to define clearly what it is; we look for a second observation and then construct one or more hypotheses to explain these observations; next the most likely hypothesis is put to the test by experiment and if it survives intact we can begin to believe that we may have discovered the true explanation for our observations. But we can go further. From our tested hypothesis, the likely explanation, we can make predictions and these predictions can be tested artificially by experiment or evidence for them sought in nature. If the predictions turn out to be correct, we are more justified in believing in our hypothesis, but never to the exclusion of the evidence. We have discovered new knowledge, not empirically known before, which can be added to our present body of knowledge: we have progressed.

Sir Karl Popper,[39] one of the foremost thinkers of our times, disagrees with this popular philosophy of scientific method. He argues that none of us start from scratch, we do not make an entirely new observation on its own because we are already biased by what we know, and to make an observation we have to know what to look for. What we do is to pose questions, which we ask because we are dissatisfied with the current explanation. Research is asking questions, but as Bronowski[7] pointed out, that is the most difficult part. Sometimes people are unable to phrase the question at all and on these occasions it is clear that there is no research project to be investigated. Do you want to solve problems or create them? In research we have to do both, but above all we have to learn to recognise a problem (and recognise those occasions where none exists).

Popper believes that knowledge advances only through criticism; that, logically, however many verifying observations we find, we cannot make a universal declaration of truth because there is no such thing as absolute truth (if there were then it would have to take account of all observations made in the future) and that an hypothesis can best be tested by systematic attempts to refute it. He states that, in logic, a statement can be conclusively falsifiable although it is not conclusively verifiable. He goes further and argues that our hypothesis should be formulated unambiguously, that is as specific as we can make it, so that it can be exposed as clearly as possible to refutation. We therefore have to ask a well-defined question and not a vague one if we want a worthwhile answer. "This alone challenges us to think of things which, so far as we know, no one else has hit on".[39]

We may discover a new problem, but growth of knowledge proceeds from problems and our attempts to solve them. Moreover, our solution to the new problem may go beyond present knowledge, and therefore require imagination because what we call knowledge is permanently provisional.

Popper's view of scientific method, so different from that generally accepted, runs like this:-

● A problem exists because we are either dissatisfied with the existing hypothesis or with the expected predictions. All our observations are made within a framework because we are biased by experience and what we think we know.

● There follows a proposed solution, a new concept which we make up using our imagination and our personal analysis of events.

● Then comes the deduction of propositions, which are testable, from our own new concept (the IDEA). The more precise the information we want to derive from our proposed solution, the more testable it becomes. We should always have more questions than answers (the professional researcher finds this the most challenging and most frustrating part of his job), because the most probable explanation goes least beyond existing evidence and so will take us the least far in the discovery of new knowledge.

● Now come the tests, which include observations, experiments and attempted refutation. Popper believes that falsification, in part or in whole, is the anticipated fate of all hypotheses; certainly the mortality rate is colossal even though we all crave to be right in our idea. But, if the hypothesis is falsified it opens the way to replacement by another with greater explanatory power. Falsifiability is the criterion which distinguishes science from non-science; it does not deny that unfalsifiable things may be true. Nor does it state that non-science is nonsense.

● Finally, we have to establish a preference between competing hypotheses. Our preference should go to the hypothesis with the higher content of information (the least vague), for that which provides a solution to the problem that interests us, for that which is compatible with all known observations, for that which will encompass previous hypotheses. A tall order, but it narrows the choice considerably. As Popper remarks[39]: "All organisms are constantly, day and night, engaged in problem solving". His view of scientific method, so different from the classical concept, is more practical than the orthodox and in medicine it is recognised by the discovery of new diseases which have failed to live up to the explanation for the old.

More importantly, Popper allows for two undefined elements, luck and chance. Both play a large part in the art of discovery of new information. Both depend on the imagination and mental receptiveness of the researcher: both are difficult to define but easy enough to recognise. Popper emphasised the importance of criticism because he believed that every hypothesis should be open to criticism. The scientific method is a discipline which helps to fit together portions of the truth even though we may not have appreciated the whole. The solution to one problem may well be a new problem, but is never the same as the original; on the way, we have learnt something new about where the difficulties lie and what is required for a solution.

CRITICISM

A major function of the brain is to organise the individual parts of our experience into a coherent whole to establish general principles for use in our environment. We commonly assume that in this process we approach experience without any prejudices in favour of one way of organising its parts rather than another. We think we are unbiased and rational, but reality is different. Experience, however, is a continuous whole so that the mere breaking up into parts is arbitrary and involves identifying particular features as being the significant ones for our immediate purpose.

This process of selection is also a process of simplification, which carries over into our research. We want to find something, make some discovery, but what is the least we will settle for? The simplest view of truth. Simplest because that will be the easiest and quickest to write about and pass on to others. We look for simplicity and directness. Yet reality is complex and the more simplified a system is the less close its relationship to the external world, and the less reliable it is as a basis for action intended to change that world in a particular way.

We improve our understanding of the world partly by observing and reflecting on the results of our own actions, but mainly by formulating our understanding in language and communicating the sentence, thus framed in speech or writing, to our fellows. We thereby open the way to rational discussion, because vague impressions cannot be criticised as words can. Two conflicting tendencies are to be found. The first seeks to extend critical discussion with a view to reducing discrepancies between the external world and our interpretation of it, in other words between fact and thought. The second seeks to avoid, or at least limit, discussion of certain interpretations, to cajole rather than convince. The first is scientific method, the second is the area of propaganda. F.H. Bradley noted that "we reason in general, not to find the facts but to prove our theories at the expense of them".

"The line dividing scientific method from propaganda is in any case easier to discern in practice than to describe in words".[1] Propagandists do not dispense with arguments; they simply do not offer alternative explanations. Those propagandists who use scientific method try to persuade others that their own interpretation is closer to reality than other people's; they are usually concerned to make action more effective and are less concerned with truth. "The scientist can do no more than make theory approximate more closely to truth than before because to be completely true theory would have to take into account all relevant observations, including those which have not yet occurred".[1] Scientific method encourages a plurality of sources of information, fosters various interpretations, looks for criticisms. Propaganda does none of these; it cannot afford to.

Now do you understand the importance of criticism in research? Do you now appreciate Karl Popper's view of scientific method? If you do, you are on the way to developing the true spirit of scientific method. Sadly, in your reading of published papers on your subject you will come across many that are propaganda. It is common in even the best research that a point will be reached, sooner or later, when a long established interpretation of the facts is found so difficult to reconcile with reality that even its adherents discard it. Hence some hypotheses and theories (the name we give to canonised hypotheses) fade away; others have to be aggressively refuted. But "theories are repaired more often than they are refuted".[41] Propaganda shouts down intelligence and has a large emotional element. Scientific method, by contrast, does not allow for emotion or feelings; it is concerned with evidence, interpretation, and criticism.

Criticism is central to scientific method because, without it, how can we know when we are wrong? But criticism is difficult to accept and self-criticism harder still. "The most essential gift for a good writer is a built-in, shock-proof, shit detector" wrote Ernest Hemingway: blunt and to the point, but the same applies to the good researcher. Research and writing are both creative, both depend on ideas, and, when these ideas become personal, criticism is never welcome. The right of original discovery is not the right of property. Criticism of one's own writing is a tough business and, at first, it can be painful and embarrassing; later, when you are able to delude yourself that you have written well, it is exasperating to admit you've produced work that is dull, null and void; and that you will have to start all over again; and wonder how you will ever capture such bright ideas. But if you are to develop as a researcher, the ability to formulate an idea as a testable hypothesis has to be accompanied by an ability to criticise it. In the end, of course, the only way to communicate your idea, your intuition, your imaginative germ, is to gain an understanding of every facet of the edifice which contains it, and put it into language. We think in language and we communicate in language.[48,49]

YOUR MENTOR

What can your mentor do to help you with ideas? Usually very little: you are on your own. But a mentor can and should do two things: first, he should make sure that you understand scientific method – its reason, its philosophy, and its value – because that is going to be the ultimate test of your IDEA. Second, he can ensure that you will be patient and not rush into things before they are properly thought out: make haste slowly or, as Horace put it, *festina lente* is an excellent motto at this stage.

He may tell you more. Scientific method was devised by philosophers, yet it has done little for the discipline of philosophy when compared with the enormous advances it has encouraged in physiology. Research is asking questions, based on imagination, but they must be within the scope of scientific method. Popper points out that it is unproductive to ask those vague and all embracing questions that pass for philosophy in some quarters such as "What is life?" "What is gravity?", and "What is freedom?" (one reply is that freedom is the right of the individual to choose his own form of captivity – a nice piece of word-play). The question must really be a proposal, because only a proposal can be put into practice and when that occurs it can be tested. We are searching for what Popper[39] calls "objective knowledge".

If your mentor makes you think out your idea until it becomes crystal clear to all what you have in mind, then he has done you a great favour. How will he know your idea unless you tell him? How will he understand unless you tell him clearly?

If I were the good fairy instead of the wicked aunt that is what my wand would bestow at christenings: the blessed gift of curiosity. Curiosity is the elixir.

Eleanor Bron

3

PLANS AND PLANNING

H.G. Wells[67] wrote that human history "is in essence a
history of ideas". Research is essentially an idea with a
means of testing it. Now we have to remember that
research is an eminently practical affair and that time
spent on planning and preparation, often more time than
that spent on the definitive experiment, is necessary and
rarely wasted. Indeed it is common to see time wasted on
ill-conceived and ill-planned ideas because there has been
a mad rush to get some project off the ground to meet a
starting deadline.

Ideas come from imagination, planning comes from
practical experience and action should follow the drawing
up of a reasonable plan. When you have written down, in
as much detail as possible, what you intend to do you do
not yet have a perfect blueprint for action. As Eliza
Doolittle said: "Words, words, words. I'm sick of words.
Show me". Now is the time to put the plan into action, to
discover if you have got it right. This is the step, from
theoretical contemplation to practical activity, that many
people funk. They begin to think up reasons for more
information, more planning and forget that famous
dictum: why think, why not try the experiment?

PROJECT, PLANNING: THE KEY GUIDES

Plans, planning, project and protocol; the four Ps, but
what do they mean? They mean that your IDEA now has
to be developed into a practical proposition – two more Ps
and by far the most important – which you yourself, with
or without help, can accomplish to find a useful product at

the end of, say, six months. It can be a daunting prospect, but with a little foresight all will be well.

Projects must have a clear start and finish. Examples are the construction of a dam, the building of a hotel, the implementation of a computer programme; the list is endless but all have one feature in common, that projects are normally specific and complete tasks within a precise time. A research project falls within this general definition, and there are seven different aspects of planning to consider. In looking at different projects, large and small, there are common points, or guide lines which require study; they are based on good management principles.

First, define the project. If we do not define what we are trying to do, we are unlikely to achieve it. In my experience, this is the rock on which most research projects founder. You have to think out and talk about your project until you are quite clear in your own mind what you want to do. This takes time; it can't be rushed. Some people say "I want to do research", but they would not say "I want to build a house" without expecting to answer a lot of questions. In many ways the greatest value of a mentor is to ask questions so that you are forced to think about the answers and so clarify in your mind the proposed project. The object must be to continue to question, search and identify until we are satisfied and confident that we have all the facts that are possibly available at the time. We must also be prepared for change in our definition because research does not stand still: our requirements or priorities may change, technology may improve, or our environment may alter.

Second, look at resources: finance, human effort, equipment, space, other facilities. There is always a compromise between what resources are desirable and what can be funded. Time is always too short and resources too few!

Third, we have to consider not just the time required to

carry through the project but also the time needed to collect together our resources. We therefore have to work out a starting date for the project, and the finishing date has to be realistic.

Four, how reliable are the research methods: are they proven and acceptable techniques or new and unpredictable? Many a promising project has slowed to a halt because the methods were previously untried.

Five, how much will it cost? In commerce, price minus cost equals profit. In research, project plan minus cost equals publication. It is common for research to falter or fail because the cost of continuing it, and so being able to finish, is too great.

Sixth, and last, we will need to measure two things: first, progress of the research against time to monitor that all is going according to plan: second, we need to measure the research data, the results, and have some idea of the volume of that data and how to handle that amount. We need the help of statistics but have to consider who will calculate and analyse them, by what technique and whether we need the services of a computer. As a general rule, the novice who must have a computer to handle his data is in deep water.

Having considered these six key guides we should now be able to say with Rudyard Kipling:

> "I keep six honest serving men,
> They taught me all I know,
> Their names are What, and Why and When,
> And How, and Where and Who."

Problems that occur later are usually due to the inability to answer one of these six questions at an early stage of planning because it had not been thought important.

Planning is the most important part of a research project. It is also the most time-consuming and usually the most exciting – indeed so much so that it is easy to become a permanent planner and never achieve anything. How-

ever as the old Army motto states: time spent on
intelligence is rarely wasted. But planning is largely
"management by objectives", which simply means that
the aim of any research is stated in advance. It is too easy to
change your mind half way through the work and end up
nowhere. The plan must be thought out well and in detail
because poor planning can easily become research by
improvisation. That is the wrong way round: the
researcher must hold the initiative and not be overtaken
by events. Disorganised research never turns out well,
never gets published, but may keep its originator happy
for years! To make sure that you will do what you plan to
do, write it all down as a protocol.

HOW TO WRITE A PROTOCOL

Tidy people often have untidy minds and untidy people
may have tidy and disciplined minds. The test comes in
writing out the protocol. Some of the best researchers in
the business work from desks that look like compost
heaps, but this is not an imperative for talent. I can only
speak from experience, that the man who neglects his desk
often puts that energy into his laboratory. It shows in his
research, and that is what matters.

The word protocol causes confusion to members of the
public because the researcher bandies the word about,
knowing what he means yet never bothering to define it.
Anyone who looks up the word in a dictionary will be
surprised by the variety of meanings. The word comes
from the Latin "protocollum", the first page of a volume,
the flyleaf glued to the cover and containing an account of
the contents. There are four more and separate meanings.

First, it can be the original note or minute of a
negotiation or agreement drawn up by a notary and duly
attested, which forms the legal authority for any subsequent deed.

Second, it can be the original record of a treaty or other diplomatic document signed by both parties to be embodied in the formal treaty.

Third, it is used to indicate the formulary of the etiquette to be observed by the head of state in official ceremonies: perhaps the best known meaning for most of us.

Fourth, protocol means the official formulas used at the beginning and end of a charter, as distinct from the text which contains its subject matter.

So what does it mean in research? It means all these and more. Note that three of the above meanings concern formal as opposed to informal events. A protocol is the formal document of the plan for a research project; it sets out the idea and the means for testing it, the time and the money this may require, and what is to be expected.

In research, the word is used in a rather special sense and for one specific use: it is the written plan of procedure, the prescription for action[10,60,66] When writing a protocol, you will in effect be writing the basic structure of your research project. The final draft will be put to various uses: as a personal guide, as evidence of intent when applying for a research grant, as an archive of what you did and how you did it. It will be your "rule book". Peter Ustinov who joined the Tank Corps so that he could fight his war sitting down, said that the Army taught him one thing: it is just as difficult and hard to do the wrong thing as the right (his autobiography, "Dear Me", 1977). "One of the distinguishing attributes of a good research worker is his ability to find good questions to be answered. A good question is one whose answer will matter".[38]

The title should be explanatory of the project, not the snappy title that you imagine as right for publication. Include the names of the principal investigators, any associated investigators or advisers, and where the work will be done.

The introduction describes the need for the research. Try to give two or three relevant references to other work to support the need for your project.

The aim of the research should follow naturally from the introduction. Make it short and clear. Better still, put the aim into one sentence.

Statement of the problem as you see it and your overall plan of study. This is really a summary, enlarging the introduction which now has become a question, and describing your plan to answer the question but omitting fine detail. This paragraph attempts to focus on what you wish to do.

Details of methods must include a description of the exact procedure, because you have to show that your proposal is practical, that you have thought of possible obstacles and have likely solutions, that your plan is geared to gathering data. The population to be studied, the sample, laboratory methods, questionnaires, and organisation of any field work should be described; when discussing the population and the sample you should justify them both, including the particular sample size chosen.[32,53,55] In this context, tables and charts may help to get your message over clearly.

The stages of the various procedures during the research, or different phases of the investigation, should be listed and a note made of what is to be achieved at each. A project that can be divided into stages has certain advantages because it becomes easier to identify difficulties and easier to find advice on how to solve them.

Analysis and interpretation means this: describe how you intend to analyse your data to answer the question proposed. Evaluation should not be a matter of judgement alone: the assumptions and justifications you intend to use must be written into the document, because either may be false.

Application of the findings. What do you expect the practical results of the project to be? What do you hope to find that will benefit you and others? Even before you start research you should have an idea of what you expect to find, but do not allow these expectations to interfere with the findings. In military intelligence, the obtaining of information is only half the story: it is the use which is made of the information that is important. The same applies to research.

Proposed schedule. When do you expect to start? How long will you spend on each stage of the investigations and why? When do you expect to finish the work?

Facilities available. Describe what is already available, such as laboratory equipment, computing, technical help.

Finance. Make out a budget of expected costs for each year of the research project, including staff, equipment, and consumables. The budget should be realistic and the costs justified by the project
Appendices will include:-

- detailed criteria for population samples, size and selection,
- tests to be applied to samples before their acceptance,
- questionnaires,
- methods of coding or identification.

STATISTICS

To provide statistics is one thing: to induce people to believe in them is another. Interpretation of numerical data is more difficult than people think, and to convince others to act on the evidence is unusual.[31,32,62,68]

Statisticians are depressing people. If you ask them a simple question such as "how many patients must I treat with this new drug to be sure that it works" and so be able to write a paper one jump ahead of the field, the reply is an uncivil list of questions which are impossible to answer. What level of significance? What degree of variation? And all you wanted was a number! What about 100, a nice round figure which we could deal with, without too much trouble? You must learn the words, the terminology of the specialty, what they mean and what they don't mean. There are many fallacies and myths. For instance, correlation is not the same as cause and effect; extrapolation is mainly crystal ball gazing and must not be taken too seriously; the words "significance" and "importance" are not the same; the volume of statistics bears no relation to the validity of the results.

These are general comments.

Another serious error is making non-comparable records, in other words not comparing like-with-like, however related things may seem to be. Commonly, sex and samples are the trouble: volunteers are rarely random, self-selection is laudable but useless, time and space are interesting but unrelated, and not cause-and-effect unless you're lucky. The failure to compare like-with-like is probably the commonest error in everyday life and in research can lead to disastrous conclusions.

The changing environment does not help. Some people are never exposed to the risks that others are and wrong proportions in a population can upset careful calculations. Then there is the problem of attributes: do we all know that we mean the same thing when we say something different, or do we imitate Alice in Wonderland with words and definitions? Prospective and retrospective data are not the same. History does not repeat itself, thank goodness. Even so, retrospective studies are the hypnotics in research: a sense of well-being pervades until reality dawns. Some journals (notably the British Medical Journal) will not publish retrospective data, and, for that matter, much material so often quoted as a stimulus to new ideas turn out to be disappointingly ineffectual. Dubious statistics are commonly caused by small numbers, but don't be taken in by the power of large numbers. If the basis is wrong, then large or small numbers play little part in the creation of rubbish. Never believe that "errors balance out" (lucky you!) and be clear about the "normal" (ever heard of it?) and percentages (a percentage of what?).

Two common mistakes creep into research so easily: the first is the failure to assess the quality of the material being collected, the input: the second is the failure to realise the fallacy of "small is beautiful" and that for some projects the amount of data to be collected is beyond one's capacity.

If data are of poor quality, either because they were inaccurate to start with or because the methods were suspect, then giving numbers (which are mathematical symbols) confers an air of respectability which was never deserved. If these numbers are then treated as valid and subjected to proper statistical evaluation we may end up with material that looks eminently respectable and difficult to refute – means, standard deviations, correlation coefficients, tests of significance with pro-babilities. And it is very easy to do: just put it all on a computer and information spews out. In computer language, rubbish "in" means rubbish "out" even if the packaging is deceptive. Rubbish in, fact out, also occurs and may be calamitous. What starts out as perhaps a useful indicator of performance soon becomes a measure of performance as "cause and effect" are presumed. How material is collected and who collects it do matter.

Some research is condemned to dealing with small numbers and there are special statistical techniques to cope with such problems. But small samples can be biased samples; two samples compared may both come from within the normal range and comparison becomes a dangerous delusion.[31,32]

FORM AND DISCIPLINE

All research, like all art, has aesthetic form; it is the most elementary, simple, crucial and exacting concern of the creative researcher. Indeed, early on, a researcher learns that the choice of form is his first concern. And form is decided by what you wish to find. It often happens that the most intriguing discoveries come not from the central plan of a project, but from lucky accidents that happen along the way – the serendipity principle. In the same way, error is part of human fallibility: "We simply guess wrong, take a wrong view, form a mistaken opinion".[40] In this context, luck in our investigation makes sense: the lucky accident fulfils a prior expectation, however vaguely formulated it was. Luck and sweat are related, because we will not recognise luck unless we work hard at our project.

Some go fishing in the great sea of life expecting the sort of catch recorded in Galilee 2,000 years ago (Luke 5.1–11). They fail to notice that they have no divine right to catch anything. Statistical probability is against them but they press on by including so many different measurements that one of them is likely to be abnormal. Much woolly research gets into the published literature because of this technique of "trawling" for data. It is to be deprecated and rarely honours its author: hence the slogan – have data, what is the problem?

If you have an idea for research how will you set about it? The deliberate decision to do it one way and not another is the slant. Let us consider only one form, the comparative trial. If we want to compare, say, a new drug or new technique with the old, how can we do so fairly and discover which is really the better?

The aim is to compare a new procedure, new drug, new method of management with standard practice. It is important to compare like-with-like which we all realise is difficult, but we do acknowledge that bias and favouritism must be eliminated. The comparative controlled trial has very wide application and has not been exploited enough. In medicine it is the principal method for measuring the effectiveness of a new drug; it could be used in industrial management, education, teaching and other professional practices to equally good effect.

Several authors have described the three stages in the development and adoption of expensive medical techniques. First, initial work continues until researchers are confident that the techniques can be applied safely to patients: even then, the technique may be confined to a few centres, not because of expense but because an interval of maturation is needed for all new ideas. Second, clinicians run trials, report them, and the technique is debated at conferences (often the early warning of mishaps is obtained at such meetings). Third, the technique is introduced into the National Health Service and general medical practice, hopefully before the technique has been overtaken by a better one. In practice, many new techniques are introduced with too little evaluation, too little research, and too little consultation, by the fear that we are "old-fashioned".

There are seven principles which must be observed if the results are to mean anything. They are described for convenience of writing as though a new drug is being tested but, with little modification of working, are applicable to all situations.

First, there must be clearly defined terms of the condition to be treated: the right of entry into the trial must be precise and specific. Qualifications for entry will not only be a named disease, diagnosed by specified physical signs, but the disease at a certain stage. Age, sex, status and social class may also be listed because we know that these play a part in the progression or regression of some diseases. The people that we allow to enter the trial are those whom we believe would benefit from a new form of therapy and that the benefits are likely to outweigh the risks. The patient's agreement (consent) is required to enter the trial, not for specific allocation.

Second, all those who qualify for entry will be allocated at random to two equal groups: the "controls" who will receive standard therapy and care, and the "treated" who in addition will receive the new drug to be tested. The process of random allocation is important. It means that every patient has an equal chance of belonging to the "control" or "treated" groups; as a consequence the results will have a normal distribution and so be analysed by conventional statistical techniques with valid levels of significance. Evidence of random allocation can be provided by measuring the height and weight of all patients in the trial: the mean value and standard deviations should be practically identical for the "treated" and "control" groups, data with little bearing on the main point at issue but assurance of good experimental technique.

Third, the new drug should look like the standard drug so that those administering treatment do not know in advance what the patient will be receiving and so cannot inadvertently or deliberately influence the results.

Fourth, both groups must be treated at the same time and under practically the same conditions: time is an important variable and environment can play some part too.

Fifth, all patients are cared for in the same way and under the same conditions. The same symptoms and physical signs are recorded for all patients. To this end it is usual to devise a special form on which data are recorded in the form most suitable for analysis later.

Sixth, the observer recording data after treatment should preferably be independent of the person prescribing treatment.

Seventh, analysis of results should be made by an independent person who has had no contact with patients but has taken part in the statistical planning before the trial started. Many people conducting trials fail to appreciate the numbers required to be entered before analysis is possible. As a consequence, favourable "trends" are thought of as "nearly significant" statistically, which is rubbish.

These principles are strict – some think unnecessarily strict – but for one good reason: to eliminate bias and ensure fair comparisons.[10,12,35,60] There are special statistical techniques devised to overcome the failings of inadequate numbers or the difficulties of disguise, but they too need critical appraisal; in some instances comparative trials are not possible, too difficult to perform, or not considered worth the effort.

THE IDEAL RESEARCH PROJECT

Is there such a thing as the ideal project for the newcomer to research? Probably not, but the following six points come close to defining it because the perfect beginner's project to start on would include:

● A well defined question to which an answer seems possible within a reasonable time. The answer should be based on clear and unequivocal evidence, the hypothesis testable by a fairly simple experiment.

● The methodology should be clear and the techniques to be used should have been proved to be reliable and be well-established. Accurate measurement of the object searched for is highly desirable. The plan should be specific, detailed and feasible.

● The whole should be within the competence of the researcher and require the minimum of expert help.

● The whole should be such that the work can be repeated easily by another of more experience, greater reputation, and more senior judgement so that the project is readily accepted by the profession, trade or occupation of those whom it concerns and who stand to gain by it.

● Cheapness, because so often in research cheapness means efficiency and efficacy and time will not be spent looking for finance.

● The project should open up the subject by posing further questions that could be answered by further research, the idea being to uncover problems that were not recognised or not thought of before! It should be interesting to explore and the results important.

A good project is a mixture of a good idea, good planning and organisation, a bit of luck, an element of chance, and a little flair at the right time. The correct mix may provide the perfect project, but such things are rare and mostly we have to accept and put up with imperfect projects. Yet the best news of any project is that "all went according to plan", a simple vindication that planning was worthwhile.

The imagination plays a far greater role in our lives than we customarily acknowledge, although any teacher can tell you how great an advocate the imagination is when a child is to be led into a changed course.

Dorothea Brande

4

READING AND RECORDING

Taking up research means that you will have to read more, more deeply, and more widely than ever before. Moreover, you will have to make a written record of all that you read and do. Both these activities – they should never be chores – are for one specific purpose: to advance the research project.[3] Reading will have four purposes.

First, to keep up-to-date in your own field of daily work. The minimum requirement is about four textbooks a year and a couple of journals read weekly or monthly. Curiously, in many professions, some practising members never look at a book or journal from the day they qualify: research for these people will be a foreign language impossible to master. They are the new illiterate: they know how to read but do not.

Second, to dig deeper, to learn more about the subject of your chosen research. Read journals, as many as relate to the project, but start from a textbook dealing with the subject to uncover key references.

Third, to keep up-to-date in allied subjects because here you may discover a useful tool to apply for your own benefit, or find a problem parallel to your own and with its solution.

Fourth, to keep abreast of advances in other disciplines so that when you meet people from these disciplines – as you surely will, if only to pick their brains – you are not completely ignorant of the goings on in their world.

In addition, you will read for relaxation. Browse among the shelves in your public library, to take out a non-fiction book on a subject you would not normally have thought of even picking up. If you get bored with the volume or the subject matter, return it to the library and try something else. Finally use fiction as an important area from which to learn how to write well. Try to pick authors who savour the English language and who treat words carefully.

Reading is a skill and like other skills quickly rusts from disuse. So, read daily in bed, bath or bog, or on the bus travelling to work: a book is much the most portable form of knowledge we have. How to keep up-to-date in your own discipline and how to dig deep in your special subject are the two most important reasons for reading: both take time and effort, and the time has to be found.

Most would-be researchers are bookworms, and many of them are fanatical about books and libraries. A love of books is part of the research life, but there is often a deep distaste at the idea of dissecting a book for style, for construction, for truth, yet we have to find out how the author has handled the problem he wrote about and to look for falsity, assumed or deliberate. That is one aim in reading a book, but the commonest by far is to obtain unvarnished facts, sometimes knowledge, rarely wisdom. There is a danger attached to searching a library. If you like doing it, then it is easy to kid yourself that you are "working" buried in a book, when perhaps all you are really doing is escaping from the project in hand. I speak from experience.

THE LIBRARY

A great many profound secrets are somewhere in print, but they are most easily detected when one knows where to seek. On most subjects there is an enormous amount published already. The difficulty is to know where to look for it and to reduce it to a form that will be intelligible for the purpose in hand, whether that purpose is securing a doctorate, overthrowing a widely-held theory, or just seeking support for a first project.

The task of the researcher is as much editorial as

original. The gaining of knowledge may be the primary
task but it is equally important to be able to transmit that
knowledge; the major problem may well be to condense
information, as a preliminary to dispatch. First, we have
to gather information, and a library is the place to seek
what we want.

There are two sorts, the general and the special[44,64]. You
will need both. You will also need to learn how a library is
set out and then learn the oddities of those libraries that
you constantly use. You have to be like the policeman on
his beat: you must know your territory and short-cuts
because you may need information in a hurry. Besides,
you will become more observant (I keep on writing in the
future tense, but your future concerns me; no one ever
learns enough in a lifetime, so the urge to learn more when
the opportunity arises must be paramount) because other
items will attract your eye and start your imagination
going.

First, examine the public library in your home town. It
is probably well appointed, warm and comfortable, has
300 reference books, including volumes of an
encyclopaedia, desks to sit at and write in the quiet,
perhaps 30,000 fiction and the same number of non-fiction
books. In addition, for a few pence, eager librarians will
order books for you to take out on loan. So how much use
do you make of this wonderful facility?

Popping in to change books on a Saturday morning is
what other people do. You are going to get the most out of
this resource on your doorstep. Do two things: first make
the librarian your friend by saying what you want. Tell
him a little of your research, what it means to you, what it
might mean to others. Second, learn the Dewey decimal
classification, because all non-fiction books will be
allocated shelf-space accordingly: fiction, of course, is
filed alphabetically.

The Dewey decimal classification is a general scheme
covering the whole field of knowledge and divided into ten

main classes, 0–9. Further subdivisions are made by adding figures to the right of the main number so that it allows indefinite expansion. For instance: 6 is useful arts; 61 is medicine as a discipline; 612 is physiology; and 612.1 concerns the cardiovascular system; 612.12 is a heart disease and so on. It is easy to follow, but related subjects can be widely separated. The main "key" is usually listed at the end of the library shelves and by searching alphabetically you can discover the relevant number and then search along the shelves until you find the text you want.

Britain has a large variety of specialised libraries. Morton[43,44] devotes a chapter to this subject which is of concern to the beginner: where can he find and read the necessary books? The answer is vital, but the choice is surprisingly wide. In medicine where books have been collected for 500 years the list of libraries is impressive: the medical corporations; the Royal Colleges of Surgeons, Physicians, and others, in London, Edinburgh, Dublin; medical societies, of which the Royal Society of Medicine, London, has the largest collection of books and journals; most medical schools and teaching institutions; some nurses libraries are particularly well stocked; research institutions; pharmaceutical companies; postgraduate medical centres, attached to most hospitals; department libraries; personal collections. There are also lending libraries by subscription (such as Lewis's in London) and the British Library Lending Division at Boston Spa, Yorkshire and the Science Reference Library, London.

CRITICAL READING

In research, reading and attending meetings are the chief methods of what in wartime is called "intelligence": information of value to you, either now or in the future, and absolutely vital for success. Interpretation of what you read is important, but the real need is to be critical. How do you know if you are reading rubbish? It is not as easy as you might think.

When reading a publication of importance to your work, examine what has been put in, look for what has been left out (the obvious and the necessary), then ask yourself these four questions:-

1. Are the conclusions justified by the evidence supplied?
2. Has the author presented enough material?
3. Are the techniques used above reproach?
4. Are the arguments logical?

There are many other questions to ask but these four are quick and essential: the answers will help decide your opinion of the work.

Every research paper has a central theme, like a thread running through a tapestry, and a central assumption, which may be an error. Try to discover both. The first will tell you how the author thinks, whether he has preconceived rigid views that will ignore data, or flexible views that can be redirected by data that may be unwelcome. The second may provide you with a research project that lets in light to an area previously obscure. Yet critical reading requires concentration, and concentration depends on several factors apart from the comfortable and quiet surroundings that most people expect: motive, interest, intention, understanding, prior knowledge of the subject, the readability of the writing, its rhythm, and personal fatigue have all to be taken into account.

The ultimate test of the value of reading lies in its comprehension: if you do not understand what you have read you have wasted your time. But the essential question – with so much reading required in research, how can one do it? – has to be answered. The answer is: first, make time to read; second, develop a variety of reading techniques and a facile ability in their use.[15] Reading is a skill that requires constant practice and a certain amount of incentive to do better.

The ability to read critically – it is not the same as being suspicious, but the attitude is much alike – is nowhere more important than when the author introduces statistics into his publication. Be especially wary of statistics – the average, percentages, decimal points – because numeracy does not imply truth. Statistics can be great persuaders or great deceivers.[32] This is not to condemn statistics but to indict those who use this useful tool flippantly. When you read a statistic, prod it to see what it is made of and ask some simple questions: Who says so? How does he know? What is missing? And finally, the acid test of all statistical information, does it make sense?

HUNTING REFERENCES

One of the words which will haunt you all your life in research is "references". In everyday language the word means a testimonial of goodness or the name given as one prepared to vouch for another.

You can give someone a good or a bad reference; you may be asked for a character reference; and all usually in writing so that the recipient knows who to blame. But in research, a reference invariably means the directive to a book, journal, or passage of some publication: name of the author, the journal, the subject, or the year of action all carry a special message to the receiver who can then uncover the material by a library search. Curiously, in T.V. documentaries this hunt for information is called research and the person who does this rather laborious work is accorded less value than the presenter. Don't confuse a library search with research: the search for literature is part of the job, not the whole. In research, a reference is an important brick in the building of a project or in its defence.

What makes a good reference paper? Credible technique and plan, convincing evidence, vivid description of materials and methods, but above all accuracy and relevance to your own project. Few papers are written like novels, fewer still are written in correct English, but the stuff is there and not too difficult to find in spite of the impoverished prose. And there is no deceit.

In the U.S.A. – from where else would the idea have generated? – there is a journal devoted to recording the number of times a paper is mentioned in the list of references given at the end of a publication. The idea is to produce a list of importance, a kind of "top twenty" in the journals business, but more likely the list is a record of idleness: why look further than the oft-quoted publication? Oft-quoted is sometimes misquoted and reading the original can be illuminating, but tends to produce letters of irritation from newcomers and the original author.

In spite of all that, there are "key references" in most subjects: often found in review papers, the very publications that are essential to your purpose. So what is the point of reading references? There are two different occasions and so two different purposes. The first is when you are flirting with a new idea, the second when the planning stage is underway or the work completed. How do you find the paper you wish to consult?

In the list of "Further Reading" at the end of this book I have mentioned Leslie Morton's book "How to use a medical library". It is full of useful information, but there is one snag, and it is this: there is an enormous difference between the tidy mind of a professional librarian and the untidy idea swanning around in the mind of its originator. The first demands a systematic search of the literature, the second a flash of inspiration. You will need both, but not at the same time.

At the IDEA stage (see chapter 2) if there is a textbook of recent date on your subject with up-to-date references then note those references, read them, and with a bit of luck they will lead you nicely into your subject. You may be a few years out-of-date but it should be possible to get the drift of whether your idea is worth pursuing or not. You will also discover the key words, so important when you come to consult a library catalogue. If there is no textbook available, look up your project title words in an encyclopaedia (Britannica and Chambers) for help there. You will now be at least ten years out of date, so start asking around: your friends, mentor, anyone, for a clue to the treasure hunt. If none of these short-cuts produce the desired publication, resort to a systematic search which you will have to do later anyway, even though it is a job which is nice to postpone until the research is underway and reading can be better directed; when you know precisely what you wish to find the hunt is infinitely easier, more productive, and more satisfying.

Even in a systematic search there is a choice; you can start at the beginning, the earliest days, and work forward in time or work back from now. Where you start does matter. For instance, in medicine, if you wish to do research on venous thrombosis there is little point in reading before 1968 because a new isotope method of detection was introduced then, and completely altered the rate of detection, methods of diagnosis, and knowledge of the natural history (the sort of information your mentor would have told you). Yet some plodders believe in starting with Hippocrates in the fifth century B.C. Interesting, but useless.

If we wish to consult an extensive bibliography on a particular subject we have to consult the earliest complete catalogues, compiled towards the end of the last century.

In medicine we start with the Index Catalogue of the Surgeon-General's Library, USA, 1880–95 which will provide references to a few books and several papers published up to the year previously. The haul is surprisingly small and the papers surprisingly uninteresting. We work through the next three series which takes us to about 1940. Almost imperceptibly the harvest has increased but not so the interest: at that time there were less than a dozen curable diseases, today ten times that number and twice as many new diseases have been identified. The explosion in medical literature was about to begin.

We continue with the Quarterly Cumulative Index Medicus, and in 1960 the Index Medicus but now have to consult MeSH (medical subject headings) to make sure that we will be looking for the correct word. The schism of a common language – of American–English and British–English – is clearly visible. The words epinephrine (USA) and adrenaline (GB), while the same substance, are not interchangeable. But these are minor quibbles. The fact is that words and actions are grouped under headings and we have to select the appropriate heading to be able to find the titles of the publication we want.

Coming more up-to-date we search the monthly issues of "Index Medicus" and "Current Contents", and begin to realise the colossal increase of published papers in the last two decades which shows no sign of slowing down. Indeed, because of recent advances in all subjects, some people prefer to work backwards in a library search, starting with a good review of the subject which usually provides a selection of the more important references to earlier work.

Even in a systematic search, forwards in time, you should be on the look-out for interesting tit-bits which may spark off a new idea or come in handy in other ways. For instance, finding the opening paragraph to a lecture (often the most important item because you may need to rivet the attention of the audience in the first few seconds) is a time-consuming necessity. Finding out about historical giants in your profession or calling is not just self-education, but a useful line of introduction to an otherwise mundane subject. Baron Dupuytren, the richest surgeon in Paris in his time, is remembered today only for the thickening of the palm of the hand and finger contracture, but he did originally describe ten new medical conditions which bear his name. The fashion to discard eponymous titles ruined him and even the hand condition would be called something else if we knew the cause and what else to call it. Morton devotes a whole chapter to the sources of such biographies and is well worth reading.

Finally, to complete this section, here is a list of ten sources of information where relevant knowledge may be found:-

Dictionaries
Textbooks and monographs
Journals
Abstracting services
Data books
Directories
Societies and meetings (congresses)
Vital statistics
Almanacks
Encyclopaedias

RECORD CARDS

If you carry a set of record cards around with you always – say A5 size – you will be in the enviable position of making notes of what you read from journals and books or hear from lectures or conversation, and file the material for easy recall.

When you read you will make notes because you will be gathering information for your project. But you will be doing more. You will be collecting references which will need to be recorded accurately at the end of your paper for publication, and an essential part it is. Unfortunately, however, some literature has names occurring in the text which are not to be found at the end of the paper, so that one cannot then read the source to discover what interpretation one author has placed on another's work. This is frustrating, and in the end it is cause enough to avoid consulting publications which could be important. But to have to compose a list of references after the effort of writing a good script is an added and unwelcome burden particularly when the seeds can be sown as you read. If each paper has its own card, it is not difficult to arrange the cards in alphabetical order when the time comes, punch a hole in the bottom left hand corner and thread through a treasury tag to prevent loss or disorder, and leave a note for the typist about how this information should be set out: the Harvard system or the Vancouver style are the most popular, but some journals devise their own which is labelled rather grandly, house style.

Every record card must contain four items.

First, the complete reading reference. The author's name, initials, name of journal, year of publication, volume, first and last pages, and the title of the article must be written out in full. Abbreviations can be misleading and so should be avoided. The idea of including the last page of an article is this: if it is not recorded then its absence serves as a reminder that you have not read the article, but obtained the reference from another source – perhaps a different journal, a book, lecture or conversation. All this information should be contained on the front of the card and will be set out like the "References to Futher Reading" at the end of this book.

Second, make a personal assessment of the value of the article or book that you have read – use such words as good, bad, important or essential – written at the bottom left hand corner, to tell you later which cards to sort out and consult when writing.

Third, at the bottom right hand corner, of the front of the record card, and preferably in red ink, make a brief remark to indicate how this paper has stimulated your work, altered your ideas or helped to confirm the correctness of your project.

Fourth, on the back of the card make notes of what you read, including the sort of data that will be valuable to quote later: such as tables and statements, written word-for-word and placed in inverted commas. It is also a good idea, and will save you much searching, if you make a note of where you read the journal or book and the date of reading, in case you wish to consult it again (write the name and address of the person you borrowed from, if it was not from a recognised library).

Important papers should be photocopied (books you will have to buy, but there will be few that you will need to), and a note of this effect made on the record card. But the photocopy should not remain untouched. You will read and make marginal notes, underline sentences or single words, ring tables or graphs, because if you don't you will not know whether you have read and digested the material and so wasted money by not getting the maximum value from your investment.

A bundle of annotated reference cards represents a valuable resource. You are rich in information, and like Shylock should look over and count your gains at intervals. Not all are shekels, but it is possible that one card will spark off a new idea in your head to fire your imagination and repay the effort of collection a hundred-fold.

THE IDEAS BOOK

This is by far the most important book you will possess. There are two requirements: that it is small enough to be carried with you all the time, and that you record ideas immediately they form yet review them frequently. As to size, something about the size of a pocket diary yet strong with it: plain pages, sewn not glued, and a durable soft cover of distinctive colour are the basic requirements. This is, above all, the foundation of your creativity, and for your eyes only. There are 10 rules:-

● Write down an idea as soon as it occurs; you may be anywhere when you "see the light", the flash of inspiration that can disappear as quickly as it came, hence the need of ready availability. The entry can be quite brief, almost cryptic: sometimes the essence leaks away with time to become meaningless, but on the whole the important notes that will shape the direction and intensity of research remain to preserve the original idea.

● Write the idea as a title, one to a page, at the top.

● Always date the entry: this may be important. Your bright idea may owe its origin to the brains of another, in which case you should acknowledge this graciously, or may be entirely original, in which case you can fight fiercely for priority.

● Look through the titles regularly and often. If you have an active mind, feed it in this way.

● Add notes to the "titles" as new thoughts occur, which they will, because your subconscious mind will be working for you when you are doing something else; the subconscious has a habit of producing bonuses when you least expect them. Rework ideas that don't seem right in the way that a poet will change and fidget with single words until he is satisfied.

● Transfer notes to your journal or day-book when an idea seems to be developing into a decent research project, even if you are not ready to take action. The transfer gives more freedom to add notes, because essentially the "ideas book" is a primer not the pump.

● Never cross anything out.

● Add a date, and perhaps the result in brief note form, if the idea is used by you or someone else.

● Look for association of ideas that you record; there

may be a pattern which gives you a clue to your main interest – and perhaps main talent – in the direction of your research.

● Include key references, the most important written records that you are given or hear about, on the relevant title page so that your visit to a specialist library may be that much more productive: *you* will know what publications to look up when the opportunity occurs.

In 30 years I have had two such notebooks: I call them my little black books, because they are, and I am surprised how many of my ideas culled from nowhere have found solutions: some completed, some passed to others (to become successful theses, for which I take no credit), some that I wish I had pursued harder because others have brought in the harvest which I failed to do, and many which still seem impossible. "To travel hopefully is a better thing than to arrive, and the true success is to labour", wrote R.L. Stevenson, and I have to agree with him.

THE JOURNAL OR DAY-BOOK

Research is rarely dramatic. Most advances are obtained from the continuous study of details, which singly are of little value but collectively are of great importance. Sincere but faulty observations and inaccurate recording are common; hence the need to record data in writing cannot be stressed too much. WRITE IT DOWN should be imprinted on everything you do, because memory is fickle and the word of others is not good enough.

If data are to be reliable you must rely on yourself and no one else to record these correctly. Never try to judge the importance of an event at the time; the chances are that you will be wrong, but if you have recorded it accurately you can assess its value in due course and have the choice: to discard or retain. Even the great Claude Bernard over

100 years ago always recorded the weight of the rabbits he bought in the market place, and tested the urine, and wrote it all in longhand before starting an experiment.

The day-book should be a sewn notebook, with cloth-bound hard covers, durable and convenient because you will probably end up with a whole collection of them, numbered volumes and with pages numbered, no paper torn out but often sheets added and stuck in (graph paper being the commonest).

A large diary with a day-to-a-page will do but the A4 or quarto size notebook is cheaper. Notebook discipline is something to acquire early on and, like cockpit drill for the aircraft pilot, it saves worry later as well as possibly the difference between success and failure. Here are ten instructions:-

1. Always write a date before anything else, and, if important, the time too.

2. Note who was present, who helped (in case there is to be joint authorship of a publication, or argument about claims of priority) and where the notes were being recorded.

3. Use the right-hand page for recording facts or observations from your research.

4. Use the left-hand page for new ideas, thoughts, preliminary calculations, diagrams and doodling; stick graph paper here when required.

5. Don't try to cram everything together. Be generous with space: it is surprising how much space gets filled at a later date.

6. Write in simple sentences, using short words which are precise and accurate.

7. Always use ink, never pencil.

8. Start new observations or experiments on a new page. Add headings or titles as needed, so you must leave space for these. Writing on alternate lines of a ruled book is a good idea: it gives you space to manoeuvre.

9. If every page is numbered consecutively it is easier to

add a note of referral to other pages containing similar material. Use coloured ink for these entries.

10. Transfer notes from the "ideas book" to the journal as soon as an idea begins to grow and develop. Add paragraphs of written thoughts as they occur to you, so that when you come to write the protocol for that project much of the effort has been invested and is ready for use. Add references and any stray comments that might come in handy. When the real work begins you already have a sizeable field to harvest.

The journal will quickly become one of your most valuable possessions. It is a resource which can be exploited at the most unlikely times, because much of research is opportunism, but we get so little warning of opportunities that we have to be prepared all the time. This book is the best insurance of preparation: guard it well.

YOUR MENTOR

How can your mentor help with reading? His value will be shown in three areas.

First, he should be able to give you a lead into your subject by providing the references that you must read. He may also know of papers on your subject which have been published in journals you might not have expected to present them, or in journals which are not readily available at your library. When you become an author you will begin to understand the urgency to get work published and the frustration when it is not in the journal of your choice. Even when he knows no references of value to you, your mentor will know the person you should consult for such information, and will provide the introduction.

Second, a mentor, knowledgeable and interested in your particular subject, is a valued discussant. He may even explain passages that you found difficult or confound you on passages you thought easy.

Third, a mentor will suggest that you join a journal club – a group of people who are prepared to read journals and discuss the contents with others. The value of the club depends largely on what you are prepared to put into it. My own experience has been disappointing, but others have found such meetings entertaining, stimulating and good value.

> A writer needs three things: experience, observation, and imagination, any two of which, at times any one of which, can supply the lack of the others.
>
> William Faulkner

5

ILLUSTRATIONS

Illustration is research's Oliver Twist: a delicate and neglected infant of obscure parentage, it has suddenly been claimed by various competing godfathers for reasons ranging from disinterested charity to commercial exploitation. From the art gallery to T.V., from the draughtsman to the fashion designer, each person uses illustration in a different way but for the same purpose: to communicate an idea from one mind to another. The painter communicates at literal, allegorical, emotive, technical, and symbolic levels; the T.V. producer has a simple approach with a single motto: "Don't say it, show it", which fits his medium nicely. So the first question to ask about illustration in research is: will it be for a publication or for a lecture? The two are vastly different: not even the language is the same.

What do we mean by an illustration? The dictionary definition "the pictorial elucidation of any subject", or even "illumination" (spiritual, intellectual or physical), is not enough for research where the term is applied to anything that is not text; "the action or fact of making clear or evident" is more to the point, and leads us to consider the uses of illustrations. They should not just be pretty pictures. In technical writing an illustration is a diagram, drawing, graph, histogram, photograph or some other form of communication which is neither writing, speaking nor gesture. An illustration can be immediately recognisable to the viewer or a complete mystery.

WHY ILLUSTRATE?

The aims and uses of illustration can be set to the author's advantage, to stress differences, to express opinions, and to provide a personal interpretation of data. Illustrations appeal to the artistic sense in most of us; many engineers, for example, draw and talk at the same time; they cannot do one without the other. The accuracy of a line drawing gives a certain sense of satisfaction to artist and viewer, and can convey what cannot easily be described in words, particularly mechanical parts in perspective drawings in engineering. Illustrations may supplement the text as something added to a description and not simple repetition – a flow diagram showing the order of various processes in manufacture, lock gates of canals to show how to get water over hills, are two examples – or complement the text by reinforcing what has been written. Hence we find script and diagram in the instruction manual to help us load film into a camera. We read the text, but are reassured by seeing confirmatory pictures in front of us.

Illustrations can concentrate information in providing a table of numerical measurements, and distil information even further by declaring the mean and standard deviation of those measurements. They may be used to amplify the text to reduce the chance of errors of interpretation, as in colour-coded wiring diagrams. They convey concepts to aid comprehension of data, such as the pocket diagram of London's underground train system: where to change and which line to travel on to reach one's destination is made simple, and thus convey patterns of information quickly so that the viewer receives a total concept. If it takes 2,000 words to describe the detail of the facade of a Victorian house, an illustration can convey all that, and more, in seconds. It is also possible to overcome lack of training and knowledge in this way: aircraft spotters can recognise airplanes from diagrams even when they have never seen the reality. It is a method of passing on information of concrete or abstract ideas in another form which may induce the viewer to read the text and begin to understand. Illustrations can also help to retain the reader's interest by "image recognition": children are often taught to read from picture books.

From this list it should be clear that there are various types of illustration, that there may be principles of design to consider, and that the choice of an illustration depends on what information is to be conveyed (its purpose).[54,58,59] The aims can be set out as shown below.

If the intention is to show . . .	*the illustration to use is* . . .
trends, or changes of one variable against another	graph
comparisons	histogram, bar-chart
proportions in relation to the whole	pie-diagram, pictogram
relationships to normal variables	scattergraph
location, geographical distributions	maps
relationships	exploded diagram, graph
new data, great accuracy, or statistical information	tables
movement	flow diagram, cine film
detail	magnified diagram superimposed or special photograph
gradations	shading, colours
depth	perspective drawing
representation	pictogram

To some extent there is a choice of the illustration you

select. Clearly one aim is impact, so how do you find out? By trial and error, by observing critically the product of other researchers, and by asking. The idea of "equivalents" is worth trying with illustrations: your data, almost certainly measurements of one sort or another, should be produced first as tables then decide what you wish to show and see which type of illustration will best convey the essential message. If great accuracy is needed then the data remain as tables with statistical differences, probability values, the type of test used, all added to the mean and standard deviation; but even tables can be restructured and simplified, sometimes even presented in two parts because overloaded tables are as common in research publications as they are in railway time-tables: both tend to provide more than you need and are irritating to consult.

The advantages of illustrations are fairly obvious. Information can be taken in at a glance: it may be conveniently condensed as in a railway time-table; there is a choice of signal (numbers in tables, words on charts; lines on graphs and diagrams; shapes as drawings, photographs, or recognised symbols; colour, groupings or spacings) and many are international currency in that they do not need language to convey meaning; it is also possible to produce three-dimensional shapes, tract directions and flows on suitable maps. They provide more impact than text on the viewer and are often remembered long afterwards.

The disadvantages are less often appreciated. It is easy to overload an illustration, to cram in all the detail that you wish the viewer to accept and so appreciate how clever you have been to collect it. The diagram may repeat what has been described adequately in the text, or worse still the viewer looks at the diagram and fails to read the more informative text. Diagrams are easy to understand but they lose precision and accuracy in the transfer from numerical information: bar charts, histograms, pie charts and even graphs suffer this loss. Hence illustrations may convey false ideas, deliberate or accidental, and their construction needs considerable skill and thought.[58,59] There is a requirement to understand the construction of an appropriate illustration because the commonest reason for its presence is speedy interpretation. The adage, "one picture is worth a thousand words" only applies when the substitution is true.

PUBLICATION OR LECTURE?

Illustrations may be used for a lecture or a published paper, but they are not the same in design, detail, or duty. Oh yes, the duty of both is to pass on information but there the similarity ends or, more correctly, should end because some people have the lazy habit of getting the illustration right for the paper and using the same in a lecture. Lecturers with bad memories may forget to have a slide made of the original art work and copy from the publication, which naturally includes the legend and the figure number thus emphasising their ignorance of the difference between these two media.

The illustration for publication must be accurate, detailed, informative in its own right, precise and of professional art standard. Anything less and it will be rejected by the journal editor or redrawn by another artist who may well miss an essential point and so misrepresent you for all time. The number of illustrations is usually limited, even though I am frequently told that line-drawings to print are no more expensive than text. The illustration should be self-explanatory, supplementary to the text, and eye-catching (David Ogilvy, a successful advertising man, said that "the purpose of an illustration is to telegraph the message to the reader". True, but in the published paper you want to hook your reader: your contribution must stand out from the masses, be noticed, and be read, and an attractive illustration will do this for you.) Published illustrations may be studied at leisure, copied and dissected to try to reveal more than is apparent.

For a lecture, illustrations are quite different; indeed we call them visual aids. The best visual aid by far is the lecturer himself, the one who speaks words that entertain, inform, and educate his audience. He uses more than words: he moderates his voice to convey emotions attitudes and emphasis, he uses gestures to reinforce his message and make the whole thing a live performance. The audience probably come to see him, hear what he has to say, and the visual aids he uses must not detract from the flow of words and expressions but complement them. Hence visual aids give fast information, are not detailed, may be purely diagrammatic to pass on conceptual or abstract ideas, and supplement the personal touch (often literally in the design of the illustration) which will hold the attention of the audience. Such visual aids will not be self-explanatory because they require the presence of the speaker to complete their meaning and convey the message.[11]

There are three main methods of using illustrations in a lecture which we must consider in more detail because each has advantages and disadvantages, yet all can be used on the same occasion: they are the blackboard, the overhead projector, and lantern slides.

THE BLACKBOARD

The blackboard or chalkboard, because not all are black but all use chalk, are cheap, common and convenient, but in modern lecture halls often surprisingly poorly lit. It is the speaker's friend, so get used to thinking with a piece of chalk in hand, and learn good techniques.[11]

Hold the chalk firmly between fingers and thumb and write with the side and not the tip. Hold the chalk low down near the business end otherwise it will break when you start to write, and write big. Write in bold, thick lines. Use white chalk, and colours only when essential to provide contrasts; limit colours to red, yellow, green on a black board – because all those other delicate colours will not stand out or be seen by people at the back – and don't overload one drawing with colours or details: make two if in doubt.

Always remove an illustration as soon as it has done its job. Write words never sentences, and place them so that they can be retained to provide a summary, but if you have to write a sentence then stand with the feet well apart and write at arm's length so that when you write words across the board you will keep them on a straight line. Print if your normal cursive hand is almost illegible. Look at your own diagrams from the back of the room during rehearsal to make sure that they are visible and the wording legible. Finally, always use the blackboard to explain concepts during question time and if the questioner is not satisfied with your answers invite him to come and draw on the board.

When you learn to use a blackboard correctly you will also instinctively learn about simplicity and neatness. Hence you can use a blackboard to mesmerise and convince your audience: you can build up a diagram as you speak, and so maintain interest: you can create a diagram in front of an audience so that each member feels that he can do likewise: you draw, keep diagrams simple, and write key words only, to save time and effort.

THE OVERHEAD PROJECTOR

This instrument is common in lecture halls and does not require the room to be blacked out. Usually it is sited off centre so that projections are always skew and not easy to get right: the easiest solution is to have the projector in the middle of the stage and the screen sloped down towards it (by tilting the upper edge of the screen downwards – not easy) until images are square, but you do have to watch that your head is not in the way. The overhead projector is an extension of the blackboard, in a way, and with several advantages.[11,51,54]

The speaker faces the audience; colour can be added to drawings, cheaply; illustrations can be prepared in advance and used many times, and x-rays usually project well. Illustrations can be superimposed to build up a diagram – if in cardboard frames the lugs make accurate superimposition easy – or the reverse where frames can be removed to uncover underlying structures. This overlay technique has many uses. Some animation, or the impression of movement is possible to imitate by skilful shifting of an overlay.

Diagrams can be "added to" with coloured transparent inks to give spontaneity to a prepared drawing and items pointed to with a pen, or better still a small pointer laid on the transparency to avoid disclosing any nervous tremor. The overhead projector is a cleaner instrument to use than the blackboard, and because clear film can be rolled on, the speaker has about 20 metres of space for his illustrations, (which can be tables, words, diagrams, charts and graphs) and at the end of his talk the whole can be reversed so that he can summarise quickly from them. At question time he can refer back to his data at will. He controls the pace of his own illustrations all the time. Because the screen is usually 6 x 6 feet or smaller the audience must be small and the lecturer can develop an intimate relationship with that audience because he can watch for feed-back all the time.

Finally, this projector allows the speaker to unfold his message by uncovering words on a prepared list. Masking is a useful technique for creating interest in the audience.

Using a sheet of ordinary white paper the lecturer can mask the whole transparency and so reclaim the full attention of the audience: by moving the paper he reveals the teaching points one by one. But he alone can read the text through the paper and can thus appear to be in complete control: he can discuss the next item before uncovering the next line of words, whereas on a blackboard he would have to remember what to say, then speak, turn silently to write, and return his gaze to the audience before continuing. In much the same way, the speaker can take an instrument or object from his pocket to lay on the projector to provide an informative silhouette without the need to make a drawing.

SLIDES

The day you discover slides you will think that one of the main problems in talking to others about research – how to put over the maximum information in the minimum time with the greatest impact – has been mastered.[11,18,21,27,28,45,54] In fact, you have now added three major risks to your simple talk. First, the danger that you will try to tell all you know by putting everything on slides. Second, that you will fall in love with your slides and talk to them instead of to the audience. Third, that you have involved another actor in your performance, the projectionist, who may be a greater clown than you by showing your slides upside-down, in the wrong order, or not at all.

From this, it is clear that when using slides there are rules: do's and don'ts; there are ten of each.

The ten dont's   Never – well, that's a relative word but break it at your own risk – overcrowd a slide: the maximum number of characters (and this includes spaces and punctuation, so remove the latter when you can and don't bother with full stops after statements that obviously require none) should be 60. Limit yourself to 20. Don't be afraid to use 2 slides where others use one. Never back-track; if you want to refer to data on a previous slide have a duplicate for that moment of recollection in your oratory: better still highlight the relevant data on the "duplicated" slide (boxed in, coloured, bolder lettering – there is scope for personal artistry). Never use words when a picture will have more impact. (T.V. producers are taught: don't say it, show it.) Never write whole sentences on a slide (if you do the audience may wonder why you need to be present as well!) but use key words and "star" important items. You can use word-slides to slow down the reader: put the first statement, abbreviated in length, on the first slide, the second statement on the second and so on, ending with one slide containing all statements as a summary of what you have talked about.

Remember the Legibility Index. If you can't read your own slide at an arm's distance, no one else will when it is projected. The size of legible lettering – and there are many formulae – will depend on this guide: screen height divided by the distance of the audience from that screen (the man in the back row is the important person) must be 8 or less, providing the projected slide fills the whole screen. Hence small screens and large halls rule out the use of slides before you even project them and start apologising.

Never ignore your own slides: if you do the audience will quickly get the message and follow suit. Look at every slide, refer to every slide, and point to the important features. Do not turn and talk: turn, point, return to face the audience and recommence talking. Important data can be referred to if you have a photocopy of the slide in front of you and can therefore direct the audience's attention while facing everyone. Alternatively you could have a mirror on the podium so that you know what is behind you. Never use an illegible slide, or an irrelevant slide, or a borrowed slide: second hand goods rarely command the top price and often look shoddy.

Never overdo the slides. The audience wants to hear what you have to say, not what you put on the screen and read to them. Never start a lecture with a slide. Never end a lecture in darkness with a slide unless it is very humorous, apposite, clever and follows the conclusions made from your research. This "ploy" requires great expertise, courage and luck: when it is successful it is brilliant and merits the spontaneous applause that occurs: when it is unsuccessful it can be the most ghastly and embarrassing flop of the whole meeting. Never use slides made from published work. Lists tend to be too long and diagrams too detailed. Slides must be simple to be effective. Do not use computer print-outs unless the lettering has been modified.

Never flash slides. It is possible to show 20 slides in 20 seconds but only if you and the projectionist are trying for a record. An informative slide needs a minimum of 20 seconds viewing time, and sometimes 1–2 minutes. No slide requires five minutes projection so remove slides as soon as their purpose has been fulfilled. Try not to show slides spasmodically. Even a disco fan would object to alternating spells of brightness and darkness. Show slides in groups of several, or better still as a complete series with no interval.

The ten do's Always plan ahead. The preparation of effective slides takes time. So allow several weeks to work out what is wanted, how it can be simplified and the most appropriate form for the audience. Use bold lettering, but no letter should be smaller than 5% of the total height of the artwork. Keep it simple! Use key words only, not sentences – but if you do, don't read the sentences to your sleepy audience – 15–20 words are ample. Simplify diagrams: leave out all detail. Simplify maps by using an outline. Disclose information progressively: give the aerial view first, the wide perspective, then focus down to limited detail. Take the audience with you as you speak – slides must complement what you say and at the precise time otherwise there is the conflict to listen or look – and to do the job effectively and efficiently you may need several slides.

Use pictures whenever you can, not because "one picture is worth 1,000 words" (in medicine the reverse is commoner: we call it diagnosis) but because the audience may get the message quicker from a picture than from your words, and may see more than you say. The latter is very important and may well be brought out after the lecture during discussion. Pictures must be precise. In other words, do mask the irrelevant and enlarge the relevant: disclose what is essential and get rid of the background unless this is pertinent. Pictures can show things for which apt words are difficult to find and in that event allow the picture to do the work for you and stay mute. Do use graphs and diagrams in preference to tables when you can because data may be absorbed more quickly; the brain tends to accept patterns better than numerals.

Observe the proprieties: number your slides in the top left hand corner, spot the bottom left hand corner (the internationally recognised guide for the correct orientation of each slide), place the slides in the correct order and the right way up for projection (the spot is now at the top right hand corner and facing the projectionist) in a firm, dust-free container. Always clean your slides with an anti-static cloth beforehand: any finger marks can then be blamed on the projectionist. Always show slides in a continuous series, and give the impression that you know what is coming next. Always be familiar with your slides at the peculiar angle of the view that the lecturer has of them and of which the audience is rarely aware.

Be positive in what you point out on a slide, never show doubt, disbelief or complete lack of recognition of your own material: the look of stunned surprise is quickly noticed by the audience. Always remove a slide when it has done its job. Replace it by a "filler" slide to regain the complete interest of the audience.[11] The "filler" will therefore be a muted colour, rarely a landscape and never such that the attention of the audience is diverted. The regular changing of slides may be the only stimulant to some members of the audience to keep awake and you may have to vary the pace of slide projection to prevent hypnosis of the susceptible: you can of course use slides to pace your talk but only for a short time.

SOME PRACTICAL POINTS

There are a few good books to help you in the design, execution and use of illustration, but the most practical help will come from a practising artist. Even so you may have to produce the work yourself as a DIY exercise. Surprisingly the work can be of professional and publishable standard without a great deal of effort, and the process of learning techniques is enjoyable. There is a tradition, rooted in centuries of experience, which dictates that no one hires people brighter, keener or more intelligent than themselves; surrounded by yes-men, all ideas will meet with approval and there will be no competition, no intellectual stimulation, no intelligent conversation and no imaginative new thought. In seeking illustration this negative attitude is disastrous: consult only the best, imitate only the very best and keep striving to do better. In this way your illustrations will communicate correct information effectively.[11,54] There are three terms central to efficiency and effectiveness:
- legibility: can the data be seen clearly and easily?
- readability: are the data set out in a logical manner so that they can be scanned easily and quickly?
- comprehensibility: do the data make sense to the

audience aimed at? Are data presented appropriately to the capability and capacity of that audience to understand?

Three long words and four questions which determine the impact of visual illustrations, but there are other aspects to consider.

● Buy the right camera and use it. The man who always carries a camera will record what he needs now and what he may need in the future, with little effort. Efficient photography depends on three things: a lens, light, and composition. The composition will be some aspect of the research project, the lens should be right for the job – probably one of the quality "macro" lenses which can focus from ten inches to infinity – and the light can be diffused daylight or electronic flash. Make a list of what you want the camera to do for you, take the list to a photographer for clarification and then to a dealer to provide you with facilities that you need, no less and probably no more. Then learn how to use your camera to best advantage. A tripod is usually a valuable extra.

Use black-and-white film because it is cheaper than colour, tolerates errors of exposure, detail can be enlarged simply and cheaply, and scientific journals publish black-and-white illustrations but rarely colour (indeed colour is often disappointing). The professional photographer is prepared to expend several rolls of film to obtain the picture he wants: you must be prepared to take three or four shots to find the frame you want. There are plenty of manuals on how to use film and a camera but only you can take care of the action: to record aspects of the research project, to make your own slides for a lecture, or to form the basis of illustrations for publication. Every film should be developed, examined, and some selected frames printed, but you will need a record system for retrieval of relevant material and a method of storing films.

● Colour is controversial. It must be used for a purpose and not for embellishment.

Tables, artwork and people can all be photographed on colour film and will be returned by the processor mounted and ready to use as lecture slides. It is therefore possible to put together a set of visual aids in a very short time, but you have to know how to do it.

Very few journals publish colour prints: the tints look wrong and the whole out of focus. Black-and-white prints made from colour slides are never as sharp as those from black-and-white negatives: indeed black-and-white prints and slides used where colour has become the accepted, such as for microscopy, may provide better detail and sharper definition.

Be consistent in the use of colour: red for danger, blood and blood vessels; green for safety by implication.

● Matters of lay-out are dictated by convention, the journal of publication, and personal choice. The last is important because lay-out largely determines the impact of an illustration on the reader and audience: content, as in advertising, is of secondary importance.[11,54,58] Here is a check list:

- headings, subheadings, and paragraphs in text are needed to isolate ideas and to break up the printed page,

- lower case letters are easier to read: all capital lettering of words slows down the reader; suitable lettering and wide spacing makes reading easier,

- labelling of graphs, tables, diagrams and charts, must be clear,

- framing of tables and charts can be done by margins and text and these may be more pleasing than "boxing in" by lines,

- word lists of, say, conclusions, can be set out attractively if planned with what William Blake called the "imaginative eye".

● If there is a choice of signal to pass to the audience, either word or diagram, always choose the diagram. This means that every "word slide" – the easiest way of conveying a message, easiest that is for the lecturer but usually depressingly uninteresting for the audience – has to be examined critically before projection. Even a cartoon of contrived humour may be better than a large slice of text. For publication the reverse is often true and frequently demanded by the editor.

● Line drawing is the most convenient, most easily reproducible, and most generally acceptable form of illustration in research lectures and publications. The problem is knowing how and where to draw the line. All graphs and charts should be drawn in rough on graph paper, then placed on a light box so that the definitive illustration can be drawn on plain paper yet retain correct proportions. For graphs, the vertical and horizontal ordinates should be drawn less boldly than the lines joining the actual data points; true graphs are spiky creatures, not the gentle or erotic curves that selling agencies prefer to see, unless the data really justify them, which is rare.

There are rules for line thickness and conventions for symbols which should not be ignored.[58] Many tables benefit from being drawn in rough on graph paper, so that the "feel" for the spacing required between numbers can be gauged. The art of the cartoonist lies in his ability to leave out lines as much as his skill in placing the main ones, and tables benefit from the same treatment: omit vertical dividing lines, all "boxed-in" lines, and then see how many horizontal lines can be erased and the illustration made more pleasing. Small tables may not require lines at all, so why put them in? The more lines that are left to the imagination the better the presentation.

● Shading used to be one feature distinguishing the professional artist from the amateur. Now that a variety of types of shading is available as rub-on adhesive sheets their use tends to indicate the amateur and insufficient planning. Sometimes shading is needed to distinguish objects, introduce perspective, or create impact, but the correct "grain" must be used for the job: closely spaced dots when reduced in size quickly become uneven shades of grey.

● Abstract and representational drawings often teach more than detailed photographs: they are quicker to understand, easier to photocopy, often well remembered, and are frequently reproduced accurately by a viewer long after they have been seen.

● Style in illustration is hard to define but tends to develop with practice. The ideal style is to produce an illustration which has impact and an immediate, clear, and correct message for the viewer, is self-explanatory, tasteful, has the clean lines of the expert's touch and design, yet is simple to produce with consistency.

● Your mentor should be adviser and art critic. He will tell you which artist to consult, what relevant publications to note, while assessing the value, importance and impact of your own illustrations. Art may be a rather personal thing but illustrations have a function and if they fail in that they rarely have any intrinsic value. Never be mesmerised by pretty pictures, especially your own.

● One proven prescription for success in commercial life is this: identify a need and be the first to fill it, then be the most efficient and the cheapest; always keep one eye on the competition and the other on the look out for ways to improve the product. It all sounds so delightfully easy; in practice it is terribly difficult, and for a variety of reasons. The prescription for successful illustration is much the same. An illustration is rarely a one-off affair, nor is a commercial project as so many industries have discovered to their cost: industry, like illustrations, like research, requires continuous learning – call it education if you must – so that whoever is in charge of the outfit will become aware of the present and its deficiencies, while looking to the future and inevitable change. So be on the look-out all the time for ways to improve your illustrations and the techniques for producing them. In that way you will be one step ahead of the competition.

A QUICK CHECK: TEN QUESTIONS

One of the problems that authors and lecturers have is knowing what illustrations to put in and what to leave out: we all want to retain those with impact and omit the uninteresting, but it is not easy to gauge the reaction of the viewer. Every illustration must be examined and there are ten questions to answer and be satisfied.

1. Does each convey its message clearly?
2. Is the association between text and illustration as clear and as close as possible?
3. Do the illustrations contain the necessary minimum of explanatory wording?
4. Are the headings precise and informative?
5. Are the symbols used conventional, and are they the most suitable for the purpose?
6. Is that table really necessary?
7. Is the arrangement of data clear?
8. Are the illustrations comprehensive?
9. Are they relevant?
10. Do the illustrations reach the best artistic and professional standards?

From the point of view of an audience it is well to remember that the eye of the onlooker is in constant motion and desires to select a prime point from which to begin an ordered and interesting journey. If this initial and fleeting moment, in which the eye "questions" the object, is lost, the data or information may be shunned for ever as being boring.

Doig Simmonds

6

GRANTS

Unlike many other activities you need not tell anybody that you are engaged in research, and you don't have to elicit aid. Not in the beginning. But there comes a time when you need one particular resource, money, and will then have to learn how to get the amount required. Two of the most useful skills in commercial life are buying and selling. The important thing is the relationship between the two: buy cheap and sell dear, you make a profit: buy dear and sell cheap, a loss. Does it matter?

If you have invested your own money in the enterprise, the result certainly does matter: the first is a prescription for wealth, the second for bankruptcy. And it is not always easy to see what is happening when you are in the thick of it, as many bankrupts will tell you. What has all this to do with research? Simply, that when you receive a grant you have in effect entered into a contract to deliver what you promised in writing to do. If the grant comes from a commercial company there may be pressure to produce "confirmatory results" and the researcher begins to understand what "thirty pieces of silver" really means.

It is surprising how many people ask for a research grant as though it was a kind of passport to success. They think that they cannot start research without a grant, when all they need is a practical idea and sound advice. There are those who feel that having a grant is a status symbol, to give an aura of respectability; others wish to do research as a stepping-stone to a better position in their career. So who needs money? Research costs money. The money spent on research can come from your own pocket or someone else's. If it's your own money you may be gratifying a whim or even paying for the pleasure of your hobby: you may not be getting value for money in the ordinary sense because you can afford not to, at least for a time. But there comes a moment of truth: you cannot go on without outside support. So what can you do? Apply for a research grant of course.[4,6,10] But it's not quite as simple as that. First, you have to fill up an application form which means writing a clear protocol for a novel project, estimating the duration and costs, to make it all seem very reasonable. Second, you have to submit your ideas to outside scrutiny and therefore adverse criticism and even some bargaining. Third, you have to pick the right grant-giving body at the right time for your project. Fourth, you will be expected to submit a progress report at the end of the year, and if you don't you will be harried until you do.[14,42]

Clearly, applying for a grant is not a job to undertake lightly. Yet many do – and fail. Don't be sorry for those who submit sloppy applications: you need these failures to highlight your own application and to make sure that excellence is rewarded. Many people fill in an application form, send it to a reputable body and expect to receive all they ask for. They often fail to specify what research they intend to do. They just want the money. They are rejected out of hand, and they grumble. Do not listen to their woes.

Those who award research grants try to allocate money to projects that have scientific merit, that are capable of solution within a reasonable time, are within the capacity of the applicant, are important in themselves or would provide useful training for the applicant. Grant-giving bodies want to see success, not just as proof of their sound judgement in backing your project but as evidence that they are doing their job of dispensing money to the deserving in a manner that allows public scrutiny.

If the applicant has done a pilot project of the research he should say so, irrespective of the results. At least he has found the project possible to do and learnt how to go about it. The grant body may appreciate the information because no one likes to back a loser and most of the "unknowns" in research projects are losers!

If you can't express in language what you want to do you have not got a research project; if you can't put ideas into plain words you won't get a grant. Indeed your ideas may be unjustly condemned because they are not understood. So the first rule in seeking a research grant is simple: think before you act. The second is: apply properly. As Bismarck said: no one learns from his own experience, the trick is to learn from the experience of others. Hence, the third rule is: ask around.

APPLYING FOR A GRANT

Nowadays grant-giving bodies have their own application forms to be completed and most have this general format:-

First of all you must give name, age, address, qualifications and present post. All pretty simple stuff you might think, yet I once inspected an application on which was written opposite the word name "see separate sheet". Hardly a good start. Better, add telephone numbers and the extension or even the code-call of your bleep to show how you can be contacted as evidence that you have considered the problems of the people administering the funds. Such small details are appreciated.

If the application is being made by a group of people, include all names and status. The days when the head of the department, rather imperiously, applied for a grant on behalf of a junior have almost gone and rightly so: that was patronage at its worst.

Second, where the research will be carried out is clearly important and the names of those who provide or offer expert help must be recorded. They supply some evidence that the researcher will have supervision: many a good project can get bogged down for lack of help and this only becomes evident when the annual report announces so and then it is too late to salvage.

Third, the proposed project must have a title, for how else can we refer to it? But I must admit that in my early days there was a senior doctor who often referred to "my research" without the need to define it: no one ever discovered what it was, he had no publications to report, but he did take the idea seriously, and every Wednesday afternoon off.

Fourth, an abstract of the proposed research, which is the proposal in miniature, will allow those-in-a-hurry to grasp the main idea of your project. It has two important elements: one is the aim and objective of the research, in other words, the problem as you see it and posed as a question; the other, the research design or how you intend to solve the problem, to answer the question. Use this section to make your research sound exciting and important. Write well and it will stand out as interesting; try to make it look attractive.

Often it is easier to write an abstract with the answer to these six questions:

1. What do you want to do?
2. How do you want to do it?
3. Why do you want to do it?
4. What do you expect to find?
5. How will you know that your answer is correct?
6. Where will this lead your research?

Fifth, a detailed plan is required, and if you have followed the advice given so far, you will discover what is required in your written protocol of research. But don't photocopy the relevant pages: rewrite and condense. Include the background and purpose of the proposed research (it is always "proposed" even if you have done preliminary work to confirm that you are on the right lines), a plan of the investigations in detail because here detail really matters, duration of the research and the starting date. Give published references relevant to your project, say two to six, which an assessor can read – never two dozen.

Sixth, finance is the second most important item in any research grant: the first must be scientific merit, and the body that ignores this is foolish. Mind you, they are often related. Ask for what you need, not what you think you might need. Accountants are serious-minded people who deal in precise numbers and are apt to check your addition/subtraction/multiplication/division; and errors at this elementary level make them distrust your ability to deal with more complex problems. You have to record what the research will cost: salary, superannuation and allowances for the "hired help", special equipment, other expenses – and some damned good reasons why these are necessary.

Seventh, most application forms have space for recording details of any other grants that you receive already or any organisation to whom you have applied. I have, personally, never understood the real reason for this slot – the practice of providing such a blank space is widespread – because if the research idea and the reasons for asking for money are good on scientific merit and eminently practical, then why be curious about other income? But make a note to show your honesty about "private means".

Eighth, the necessary signatures of good faith, not of character which is rarely questioned, but that the project has the approval of your local ethical committee when appropriate (the chairman's signature is the only valid one on this occasion), that the head of your department knows and cannot later disown you publicly and get away with it, that the chief administrator knows about your research and cannot deny it to the press, that the treasurer of your institution has agreed the costs and tacitly will become liable if they are completely wrong. All these signatures help to convince the grant-giving body that you are a reasonable liability on their funds and that there are ways of taking action, by blaming other people, if their judgement is bad.

Ninth, your passport, commonly called a curriculum vitae or C.V. This is not the place to write a eulogy or an obituary. Be factual, precise and pertinent: name, age, where trained, degrees or diplomas, past experience in your profession or trade, present job, experience in research, any publications – record these correctly and if you have been the fag-end author don't put your name first, because committee members have a habit of knowing the senior author (in age) and, if his name is first, may give you more credit than you deserve. Do not include your life-history, a list of hobbies (unless very relevant), family history and all those missed opportunities: be brief and to the point. The committee want to learn if you are capable of doing what you propose: if your ideas are too ambitious you are likely to be given a chance to modify them with help and resubmit a less onerous programme. If you have made a pilot study, which supports your project, say so. Seek advice before completing the form carefully, plan what has to be included in each section – try not to have extra pages unless absolutely necessary – always have the information typed, fill in all spaces on the application form, and write good simple English.

Finally, remember this: if you are awarded a grant this will in effect be a contract, a contract to do what you said you would do, and usually to write an annual report on your findings and progress.

THE COVERING LETTER

Usually this will be brief but some grant-giving bodies interview applicants and you must discover this beforehand. There are ten golden rules in letter-writing:-

1. Draft out what you want to say in rough first.
2. Use plain writing paper or headed paper of your

institute. Type, or if you can't type then write in black ink.
3. Write clearly.
4. Keep your letter short and to the point.
5. State what grant you are applying for: it may be a good idea to use this as a heading to your letter.
6. Give all the information you're asked for.
7. Make the information you give relevant to the grant-giving body, so read any notices carefully.
8. Check your spelling and punctuation.
9. State when you are available for interview, and how you can be contacted.
10. Print your name clearly under your signature.

THEN WHAT HAPPENS?

Usually the grant-giving body will acknowledge your application, but it shows consideration to include a self-addressed postcard (application received, signed . . ., date . . .) for the research committee clerk to return: he will notice you, if no one else. If the form is discovered to be incomplete, inaccurate, or totally wrong, it will be returned for correction, but usually there is a delay of several weeks while all applications are processed for the meeting of the research committee.

Commonly your application will be photocopied so that each member of the committee will have his own, and two copies may be dispatched to selected assessors for special consideration and comments. Applications are treated in confidence, and in thirty years in the U.K. I have never known this to be broken. In my experience, assessors go to a great deal of trouble to validate the reasonableness and possibility of research projects: to make their job harder by sloppy workmanship is foolish because every applicant at this stage is a "paper candidate" for research monies.

At the research committee all applications are

considered, often debated in detail, sometimes a vote is taken, sometimes further advice is requested, but usually a decision is made. The scientific merit of the project and its originality count for most. Approval may be unqualified (you get all you asked for), qualified (the secretarial help will have to come from private enterprise), or limited (two years, not three). An efficient organisation will let you know in writing within one week of the meeting. If you have been successful then almost certainly there is an implied contract to supply annual reports on progress: some bodies give guidance on how to prepare these because a single-sheet report may be included in committee papers for members.

If unsuccessful, is there any method of appeal? In general, no. But research is a resource which has to be cultivated and encouraged, and so some bodies will recommend that applicants consult with a named person, not a referee, but someone who will help that person to reapply after correcting the methodology, enthusiasm, aims, or whatever was previously unacceptable. Most research grant bodies provide no help: the answer "no" is enough. The trouble about trying to help the refused is this: the whole thing becomes personal, quite quickly reputations are at stake and acrimonious correspondence begins and continues.

For some grants an interview may be usual or exceptional: the wise man discovers this before asking to state his case.

THE INTERVIEW

Being interviewed for a research grant is rather like being interviewed for your first job. Memories come flooding back and hopefully some of the necessary self-discipline.

First, make sure that you have all the relevant papers, a copy of your application, your own curriculum vitae, some private notes about why you want to do this piece of research, where you think your career is going and how research fits in to the scheme of things. Be prepared to defend your ideas and plan of research, and be prepared to modify the probable costs if asked to do so but never if such economies will jeopardise the whole (they rarely do, but it's a common threat). Do bring charts, photographs or illustrations if they are likely to help. Do not bring a set of slides, projector and portable screen because few interview committees have the time or inclination to settle down to your kind of entertainment.

Second, do a little homework on the grant-giving body. How was it started? Is there a special interest? What is the general philosophy? None of this information is easy to uncover, and so you will score extra marks if the opportunity arises to disclose some of it.

Third, start out early for the interview; arriving late could cost you the grant. In any case, arriving hot and flustered for an interview is hardly likely to impress anyone: we all know how busy you are, but don't wish to be reminded of the fact.

Fourth, wear the right clothes; neat and tidy rather than a snappy dresser. Try to give the impression that you are a stable member of society, a dependable citizen who will use their money well. Be the image that you think the members are looking for. You will be meeting professional people in a position to help, so why not indicate that you too are a professional?

Fifth, remember that the interview may be only a part of the process of sorting out those worthy to receive grants. You may be asked to attend again. Naturally, it is advisable to have some idea of the number of members on the interview panel, and their names if only a few. You can make a good impression by being pleasant and polite to the receptionist or secretary who greets you – it will get you off to a good start and the chairman may well ask later for her impression – and if you have to go through a closed door, knock first and then walk in. Don't sit down until you are asked to, and don't slouch: sit relaxed and upright and look alert. Speak up, don't mumble or mutter and try to act with modest confidence but never flippantly. Some candidates give jokey answers to cover up nerves; this is dangerous. Always be sure that you are on the same wavelength as the interviewer before you introduce humour into the discussion. The interviewer may prefer to make the jokes!

Remember that not all members of the panel will have the same interest in your subject, nor recognise its importance, and some may have personal scores to settle. Interviews are not necessarily civilised occasions: most are, but not all. If you give the impression that you like the members they are more likely to warm to you. Finally, when the questions are done and you are dismissed say thank-you, and leave with a feeling of confidence. Do not convey the impression you are thankful that an unnecessary ordeal is over. Try to part on good terms because you may well meet some or all of those panel members on another occasion and if they have pleasant recollections of you that will be a bonus.

HOW TO WRITE A REPORT

In other chapters there are recommendations on how to write a paper for publication, the script for a lecture, a letter to a scientific journal and even notes on composing a thesis. Here we consider report writing.[10,14,42] Clearly all these have one thing in common: the need to write well, an appreciation of style, an ability to use language effectively to communicate facts in an orderly sequence and, although pitched at a particular level in each case, brevity and simplicity are always appreciated. But there are three important differences.

First, the time to prepare a report is usually very brief:

many are wanted yesterday. The report, however, is usually written for specific persons who are knowledgeable of the subject and who will be keen to read it.

Second, the feedback is different: to a letter you usually get a reply; to a paper for publication, acceptance by the journal editor; to a thesis, the coveted university degree; but to a report, action.

Third, the number of illustrations is dictated by the kind of response you want. For a letter there will be none; for a thesis, many; for the published paper, a number limited by the editor and journal "style"; but for a report, some can be free-hand drawings, photocopies from journals or books, as well as the conventional graphs and charts (allowed to be presented on graph paper), so that the whole is stamped with the personality of the originator of the report. Every report requires a beginning, a middle, and an end. The beginning should explain why it was written, the middle contains the findings, and the end will be the evaluation of the results, their assessment, or recommendations.

What is a report? To my mind it is documented evidence that work has been done. Filed away and re-read years later, a report may become valuable evidence to be built upon in a new project even if the original data were not thought publishable or worthy at the time. It is an essential record of work and a repository of information. When we come to consider writing a thesis, one recommendation is that the author reads a review of the subject or reports of meetings and colloquia in order to place published papers in the true perspective of the times when they were written, and how people thought. A report is a written document for decision and action, and its presence simplifies both: it may disclose gaps in information or knowledge, not previously obvious, and it is a reasonable method for judging the quality of research – to a grant-giving body particularly – and may be the only method available when work is being done at a distance.

Writing a report is a challenge to a researcher to be articulate, to be accurate, and to be explicit: three features commonly lacking in many reports. The prestige of a well-written, informative, concise report should not be under-estimated: for author and institution. Writing the report, just as with any other form of writing, means thinking about the material to be included (who is it for, why is it being written, and where will it be circulated?) and making notes. There are then several stages in the craft of composition. First, outline planning, means collecting together all the material likely to be needed: opinions and fact, and references to both. Then selection of what is relevant and important to the subject title, or needed by way of explanation. A thread must be woven right through the report in the same way that a string of pearls is held together to make a pleasing article, each graded for size and quality. Arrangement comes next. The order of information can be based on logic, time, flow, comparisons, or cause and effect. There are several methods: don't confuse the reader by mixing them. Interpretation of the data should be an objective assessment because others will hold a different interpretation, perhaps to their advantage; in this section you should be acting as the expert witness, neither favouring the prosecution nor the defence, completely impartial. Finally, think about presentation. If a single sheet report is requested so that committee members may receive this synopsis with their papers, it may be wise to finish writing the report first, to be retained as the complete document, and to compose the one-page report from that.

Second, write the first draft, preferably at one sitting. Third, add, subtract, and rearrange sentences until the meaning is clear and the whole flows well. Fourth, look for flaws, of logic, in the use of language, in the data presented and in publication of sentences or information. "Every article can be improved by trimming" is a good motto. Film men always say that the best bits end up on the cutting room floor: they don't of course. Fifth, connecting sentences and summarising paragraphs should be added last to make the reading of your report easier. Distinguish these aids from "padding" which has no part in report writing.

None of this is easy. Sir Frank Whittle described the main parts and working of the modern jet engine in two sentences: "A compressor, a combustion chamber assembly, a turbine, and an exhaust pipe ending in a jet nozzle. Large quantities of air are drawn in at a front intake to pass over these organs in that order." He then goes on to describe each part in more detail. As they say in industry and research: anyone can have good ideas, it is making them work that counts. Making them work is the difficult part.[63] Some inventors don't even try but like to take credit later for ideas they didn't know how to make work. Yet even when ideas are made to work they have to be reported to others: wordcraft,[24,25,48] like stagecraft, has to be learnt and developed, for in no one is it an innate characteristic.

> Money is like a sixth sense without which you cannot make a complete use of the other five.
>
> Somerset Maugham

7

TALKING AND LECTURING

In research, it is important to talk about your project to as many people as will listen and if you are working in a research institute you will have to listen to other people's projects and problems and appear interested. You will have to learn the meaning of the word communication.

Although the process of communication is subtle and not easy to simplify, it is useful to think of it as applied to wireless telegraphy: a message is encoded by one person, transmitted over a distance on a certain wavelength, to be received and decoded by another. In a lecture, the code is language, the encoder the lecturer, the decoder is every member of the audience, and the wavelength is the subject. But the sender and receiver have to know the code, words, and gestures: so talk simply and clearly. Both must be on the same wavelength, have the same interests, and be in sympathy (the two are not the same). There must be a minimum of interference. There must be a good genuine desire to communicate, to give and receive, to speak and to listen. Listen to an audience? Yes, listen, for you will hear much. The more that experience is shared among others the better the chances of successful communication, because people in the same job speak the same language. Even so, you must check regularly that understanding of your messages and intentions is occurring. How do you check? By observing the response and the actions of the other: they should be appropriate and correct.

On radio, actors read from a prepared script and providing you don't hear the rustle of paper it can be quite life-like. On T.V. the actor has to memorise the script and add gestures to make it all acceptable. Lecturing is T.V., not radio. When the lights go down and the monotonous slides appear, it imitates radio, but it is unreal; for this reason the subject of the technique of lecturing is dealt with later, and slides in another chapter. There are, however, six different speaking occasions to consider.

First, the small informal group-discussion, a regular feature, weekly or monthly among those in the same institute or those with similar interests but from different institutions. Informality is important and successful meetings are more by way of conversation, because formality ruins spontaneity.

Second, the more formal talk, usually unscripted, to immediate colleagues on the lines of "tell us what you are doing at present and how is it going".

Third, the formal lecture at your institution, club or association: on some occasions this will be a rehearsal for the next occasion.

Fourth, a paper given at a national meeting of the research society or professional association.

Fifth, a repeat performance at an international gathering.

Sixth, as the invited guest speaker, the expert, alone or as one of the group at a symposium.

While the novice is unlikely to be called on to perform on all six occasions, four are possible and likely. It is therefore wise to learn something of the technique of public speaking[11,18,27,28,38] and the organisation of a lecture early, while the research project is underway. Your mentor should be consulted and, having had a great deal of experience, he can provide invaluable help.

THE LECTURE

One day someone will ask you to talk about your research, not always because it is all that interesting but because you could fill a gap in a programme being prepared by that other person. You may not be first choice. Don't fret about that but do think about the consequences of agreeing to talk. If your material is ready and there is ample time to prepare, then this may be a grand opportunity to excel; but if your research is not going well, there is little to report or the notice is too short – then be firm and say "no" but change the invitation to give you the chance to speak when you have something worthwhile to say: more importantly, lecture when you are ready and prepared to learn from your audience. The whole idea of talking about your research is to learn from others, to expose your idea and data to criticism by those working in the same field, to judge whether further work is needed, to listen to contrary arguments or views, and then to incorporate anything of value into your paper for publication. Many people write first and talk later. I think this is the wrong way round, if only because the printed word cannot be erased or altered; publication has a certain finality and reputations are judged thereon.

You will not be asked to tell your life story, how much you worried over the question to ask and the manner of answering it, how you overcome all obstacles in spite of adversity. No, we all have these problems and to hear the same from a newcomer is boring. You are expected to provide a shorter piece: the results of your research, a little about the detail of how you got there perhaps, but essentially what you found. In a programme of short lectures such as a "Research in Progress" symposium, you will be one of many striving for the same thing, recognition. On another occasion you may have deliberately offered your ten-minute lecture to a research society by submitting an outline, and have been chosen from among other competitors to speak.

The lecturer aims to entertain, educate and persuade his audience. But what is a lecture? The dictionary defines a lecture as "a discourse before an audience on a given subject for the purpose of instruction", which is a pity because a lecture should be a debate between two groups, the lecturer and the audience. Admittedly the lecturer has the most to say until question time, but the audience can respond in a variety of ways: rapt attention which is unusual, a certain amount of shifting about and muttering which is common, or walking out in disgust which fortunately is rare. The lecture is a contract and should do some good: either the audience goes away revitalised, or wakes up refreshed.

So what does the audience want? An interesting story with a plot spoken in familiar English and acted well. Is that all? Yes, that's all. Unfortunately, the lecturer has to write the script and perform it, a kind of actor-writer, and yet be good at both. It is not impossible if you follow these seven instructions. Do not skip a stage or try to cut corners. The advice given is specifically for your first major lecture, and is a good discipline to return to if at some future date you have to deliver a very important lecture. When you have presented more than two or three papers you will have acquired the necessary confidence that allows you the great freedom to ad lib for much of the main part, but you will still need to script the beginning and the ending: the first rivets attention, and the second finishes with a bang.

● **Writing the script**.   Spread out all the data from your research project and decide on the "plot" to present. A new technique? Important results? Interesting inferences? Unexpected conclusions? Try to pick out enough to make an interesting story to be put over within the time available for the lecture. You will not be able to tell everything, you will have too much for sure, so the job is one of selection and compression. What will interest the audience most? It's your guess; you will know roughly who the audience are, but their interest will not be quite the same as yours. The decision is a bit of a gamble, and a minor challenge to your judgement, but that is part of the fun. You will probably know more about the subject than most of the others at the meeting, so how are you going to set them alight? You are going to write an interesting script.

Every short lecture is in three parts: beginning, middle and end. The beginning, which is brief, has to do two things: introduce you and introduce your subject to the audience. They can see you and make up their minds if you keep still and don't prance around, are well-groomed and well-dressed, and have what is called a "platform presence" which usually means confidence. The opening sentence, which should at once quell the mob and hold their attention, is the most important and the most difficult to compose; it is usually completed last and often within a day or two of the final performance. The object is to startle the audience and grab their attention; unfortunately few can write "Friends, Romans, countrymen . . ." and get away with it. We have to be content with less memorable openings, yet like Mark Antony we rely on the occasion to provide us with the right words. Hence, at a symposium or conference of speakers, it is vital to hear what has gone before: therein layeth the jewel that ye seek. Take it.

The middle is the main portion of the lecture, the meat trimmed of all fat. It is the message you wish to put over and hence will follow certain fundamental rules, by using short words that punch the message home; the right word for that idea which means searching for it, but when you find it you'll know; active verbs, concrete nouns and variety in the length of sentences. Present one idea at a time, and hence three new ideas in a ten minute lecture is the most allowed. To overload the mind of another is possibly worse than trying to fill it. Finally, do try to find memorable phrases. Of all the millions of words spoken each day can you not conjure up half-a-dozen which your audience will recall with pleasure?

The end, like the beginning is composed of two parts: the conclusions made from the research and your closing remarks. They are not the same. If you have presented your research clearly, the conclusions you draw will already have become obvious to the audience. This is exactly what you want. At this late stage there should be no need to plead, to convince by statistical data, and to attempt to do so is fatal. But your final words, these too should be memorable. Plan to go out with a bang, not a whimper, which will automatically ignite spontaneous applause. Your last sentence must have the ring of truth, sincerity and enthusiasm, so that the audience feels exhilarated by your forceful words.

● **Reading and altering the script**. First read aloud what you have written, at your normal rate of speaking, but against a stop watch. If your script is within a minute or two of the 10-minute lecture time, that's good; if it is much over, say by five minutes, now is the time to cut out a large section. Reread to check if the script remains a coherent story. If you are satisfied, begin to read sentence by sentence, to discover where written English can be changed to spoken English. They are not the same language.[10] Spoken English uses different and distinctive techniques of communication.

In writing we leave a space between words so that spelling and hence meaning are easy to understand; in ancient manuscripts words were all joined together, and this occurs normally in speech. We write, "I do not know where he is", but we say "Idonotknowwhereheis" – which is called phrasing because we speak in groups of words. Normal speech of course is not a continuous ribbon of letters but the pauses are used for a purpose – as punctuation, to clarify sense or to build up suspense. In addition some sounds are changed by those that follow: we write "ten minutes" but say "teminutes", "hand carved" becomes "hangcarved" and this is called assimilation. Elision too is common, when letters are omitted in speech: "How are you" becomes "How're you". None of these can be written into your script but you must be aware of them because they will tend to speed up your rate of delivery and will give the lecture a conversational style, to make your speaking sound relaxed and natural.

Stress on words will be used to emphasise their importance, and you can underline such words in the script, but it will be the intonation of your voice which conveys to the audience those emotions of doubt, surprise, fear, delight, or sadness that no written document can ever do; indeed, the professional actor learns to use this quality to best effect early in his career. We give "colour" to our speech in this way.

Finally, note the music of speech, the rhythm, rate and pauses that make it all so tolerable and sometimes memorable. H.W. Fowler wrote:[24] "Live speech, said or written, is rhythmic and rhythmless speech is at best dead". He compared rhythmic speech with the waves of the sea, moving forward with alternating rise and fall, too complex for analysis. A comfortable rate of speaking, for listener and speaker, is about 100 to 120 words-a-minute (time yourself with a stop watch), but this depends on the size and complexity of the words, the context, and the audience. More importantly, a constant rate is dull and what you want is variety. In conversation we vary the rate because we may not have thought out our ideas before saying them and because we are watching the other for his response and understanding (feedback). In a lecture we slow down for important statements, difficult words, and speed up for the ordinary. With experience it may be possible to get the "feel" of an audience, to appreciate how much and how well they understand what you say, but it requires unusual sensitivity because the audience will not be homogenous in their knowledge of, nor interest in, your subject.

During this time of rewriting, the truly creative part of your lecture, try to record on tape and listen to the playback. If a sentence is difficult to speak it needs recasting. If the words and construction sound right then they probably are right in spite of the peculiar grammar and colloquialisms.

"Ride with the tide and go with the flow" means that words and ideas are well-matched, easy on the tongue and easy on the ear. Because the "getting it right time" can be unpredictable it is clearly important to plan well ahead of the day and use your time profitably. No good lecture was ever composed at the last minute.

● **Finding illustrations**.   If it takes five pages of print to describe a house and five seconds to take in the real thing just by looking, then illustrations can save words. The eye is quicker than the ear? Well, not always but some data are best presented visually. In general, the familiar illustrations – such as photographs, tables of numerals, and various charts – have a big part to play in developing an interesting lecture and should be slotted into the script at this stage. Every illustration, which must be referred to during the lecture, should complement the spoken word, yet never conflict with it and will be a substitute for text and not a repetition.

● **Learning the script**.   If you have composed a good lecture you will now have to "learn your lines" just as a professional actor does. There is still the opportunity to change words here and there but at this stage the play has been written and the main effort now is to polish the performance. There is still plenty to do.

First, time the whole reading at your normal speaking rate: allow 10%, say one minute in a 10 minute lecture, for mishaps without the need to worry about your allocation of time.

Second, add signposts for the audience. In writing we use headings and subheadings: in speech we use illustrations, gestures, introductory and linking sentences. Decide where these signposts will be and how they are to be indicated.

Third, learn a bit at a time: speak it aloud to listen to its sound. Does it sound like you? Is it friendly and natural? Vary the pace and pauses to discover what effect these will have on the understanding of your text; vary the speaking voice to convey the emotion that you need to accompany your words.

● **Adding gestures**.   When you stand up to lecture for the first time you will notice something unusual: everyone is looking at you. This has been called the "massed threat stare". The audience is interested in you: what you look like and what you have to say. So speak to them, be friendly, and stare back hard; more importantly search for a friendly-looking face and address your opening words to him. Then look for another and as you cast your eyes around looking for that face, people will realise that you are talking to every individual, and when you find the friendly face (as you will) speak to him alone for a few seconds. That's the first lesson in gesture: your eyes, and where your eyes go your voice follows.

But you have to be heard, so move as far forward towards the audience as you can, and that's the second lesson in gesture: body movements. If there is a lectern behind which you can hide, don't; to which you can grip with both hands, don't; on which you can place your copious notes, do so. Get as far forward as you can to the audience. "Be so near that you can lean over and take a shilling from the lady in the front row" was how Gracie Fields put it, and she knew how. She also said "speak to the back row" which means that you keep your head up. Audience attention remains with the words spoken, and so if they don't hear you, attention inevitably is lost. Finally, arms and hands can provide the most expressive gestures to the greatest number and it is natural to use hand gestures when speaking.

Gestures must have three essential qualities; they must be of the right intensity, that is that they should not be overdone or be too weak to be recognised, but must appear to be quite natural and appropriate to the words spoken yet carry an explicit meaning, and finally never be contradictory. A gesture is any action that sends a visual signal to the onlooker. To become a gesture, an act has to be seen by someone else and has to communicate some piece of information to him; a gesture should mean "observed action" and hence can be intentional and deliberate, or unintentional and reveal unexpected information. The gesture is seldom an isolated action in a lecture; it complements or supplements words and sometimes acts as a substitute for words when a gesture may be more expressive than words.

We use gestures to show friendliness, usually by a smile; to animate our speech, by emotion and sincerity; to reinforce what we say, to make greater impact, and to clarify what we are talking about. We also use gestures for speed because a single gesture can convey the whole message in minimal time and cover distances that the voice cannot. Gesture can signal a change in our thoughts and speech, to illustrate what we say as a form of mimicry because we can't help but act and mimic and symbolise our words. Anyway, you have to add gestures to your spoken script to give the impression of spontaneous interest, and convincing speech, and convey the impression that you are alive.

● **Rehearsals**.   The plural is used because there will be many rehearsals of small portions of your lecture, culminating in a dress rehearsal before the day of public performance.[11] Rehearsals are to define and refine three important aspects: impact, presentation, and timing. Any one of these can reduce the importance of what you say and mar your performance.

Rehearse a part of your script every day so that it

becomes familiar: individual words may change but the order of sentences will be remembered and at this stage should not change. You will also begin to write headings of single words on a card, in the correct sequence, to act as a prompt for your speaking. At first the list of words will be long but as confidence grows some words can be omitted and the list rewritten. Write on only one side of the card; you may need four or five cards for a 10 minute talk. Before the final· rehearsal in front of an audience of friendly colleagues, you should have had at least one full rehearsal privately, with slides, prompt cards and gestures so that you know all will synchronise and the whole lecture will flow easily.

The final rehearsal is important. It should be in a proper lecture theatre, under conditions similar to those you are likely to experience at the conference where you will deliver the lecture, and has three objectives.

First, to check the lecture time. This means that someone must use a stopwatch. If you have only a 10-minute slot, then at rehearsal accept 9 minutes but not 10, and never 11. Do not rely on being able to speed up on the day. Never over-run your time: no one thanks you for that, it is discourteous to your host, and shows an indifference to the audience.

Second, to check the clarity of argument, in other words the logic and sequence of how you present your research. This includes the connotations of words and the quality of the illustrations used.

Third, to check the intelligibility of the lecture, the words you say, the pace and intonation, your stance and gestures – all of which convey the message to an audience who may have little prior knowledge about your subject.

The dress rehearsal will provide you with one very valuable asset, the ring of confidence, because on the day you will be nervous but will be able to say to yourself that you have prepared well and know your subject. You will, of course, listen to the comments of the audience at rehearsal: there should only be constructive criticism and a little praise. You will have to decide whether to make changes in your lecture at this late stage. It means more work but is often worth it and hence the rather obvious need to have dress rehearsals at least three weeks before the lecture date.

● **The final performance**.   On the day, you will arrive well before time and "case the joint". If there are speakers before you, listen to what they say by all means, but more importantly note how they speak and how the audience reacts. Sit at the back to discover something about acoustics and visibility in the building. Time spent on reconnaissance is seldom wasted.

When it is your turn to speak you will be nervous but that is not a bad thing. You are going to speak to an audience who want to hear what you have to say; you are not going to disappoint that audience by reading a script. So what about the risks of complete amnesia, of drying up half way through, of utter failure? What about them? The risk of failure is always present in every speaker: we call it "stage fright" and it is pretty rare. You will not read your lecture but you will carry in full view of everyone a "life belt" in the form of a complete script hidden inside the programme of the meeting, and your prompt cards. You will place both on the rostrum because they are there for your peace of mind not as an exhibit for the audience. If now you forget your place during the lecture you can conveniently consult your prompt cards. Do so quite openly because the pause in speaking will seem natural, indeed the audience may appreciate it as though it was part of the act. If your mind goes a complete blank, all you need do is to uncover your script and read it aloud: when composure returns it is easy to put down the script, and as you remember your lines you will appear to be speaking extempore.

So you see, either way you can still deliver a good lecture

and put across your subject. But do something else: use the lecture to promote your product (which is yourself and your research) just as the advertiser does on T.V. by grabbing the attention of the audience. The written paper, with all those necessary but tedious details, will be published at some time in the future; the job now is to interest the audience, or more precisely to interest, entertain, and educate them, so do so, and in that order.

Two more questions remain. First, how long does your script need to be? If you speak on average at 100 to 120 words-a-minute then you will get through four to five typed sheets of A4 paper in ten minutes, but remember to deduct about 50 words for every slide shown. Hence the script is generally shorter than you think. Second, how much preparation? No lecture can be well prepared in three days; some can be prepared in three weeks, but the majority require three months to ensure comfort and time to spare. Remember that no one is interested in how hard you worked at it but only how you spoke.

The final assessment is, would you do it all again? The answer is invariably "yes", but there are some individuals who are so nervous and suffer such misery before a lecture[11] (vomiting and diarrhoea can be distressing whatever the occasion) who will give an emphatic "no". For them, good advice is to attend evening classes in public speaking[33] – held in most large towns – to learn the techniques, but mainly to gain confidence and so overcome their handicap.

STYLE

In a lecture you will be competing with others for the complete attention of the audience; you will be pleading your case publicly for the first time, so how can you leave a lasting impression on the audience? You are not expected to unveil earth-shattering new developments, just to provide a workmanlike account of what you have been doing. What you say should be new, true, understandable, interesting, entertaining, informative and with a touch of professionalism.

First, speak up. This does not mean shouting, but holding the head well up and talking to the people in the back row of the hall. Clearly you cannot do this if you read aloud, so never read but always speak a lecture.

Second, speak with confidence, which comes from practice and many rehearsals.

Third, speak with authority. Speak only of what you know, have all the facts and don't wander beyond your brief. If you stick to your subject there is every likelihood that you will be the expert at that meeting.

Fourth, speak fluently. This means having a good script, well rehearsed. The content has to be satisfying and some at least of the language memorable. Inevitably this means a lot of practising in private, rehearsal before an audience and accepting their criticisms.

Lastly, speak to time. Count words in the script, pace yourself against a stop-watch until it becomes an obsession. Audiences appreciate a good time-keeper and rarely grumble about the speaker who keeps within his allotted period. If they want to hear more they ask during question time.

YOUR MENTOR

Seek help in four areas.

First, words are the currency of research projects and publications; some words are of immense value. Of the millions of words spoken each day, many are wasted, many are not even heard and many make little difference to anything or anyone. But there are some words that are special. Some words stick, as we say; others are remembered and treasured. Your mentor will stimulate you to find the right words and to find quotable phrases, he will thus help you to develop style in speaking because uncontrolled speech has no character, but a carefully worked on spoken lecture seems spontaneous and has style. You may also need help to rid your sentences of jargon,[20] a common and too easily acquired vice in all research.

Second, your mentor will insist that you rehearse your lecture and he will make time to listen to you, possibly the greatest service and the most valuable he can give you. Try to show appreciation even if you don't care much for the constructive criticism.

Third, tips on lecturing such as timing, which is not the same as time, may save you many hours work and give your talk the professional touch so lacking in others. Timing is important. One good reason for watching T.V. repeat programmes is to ignore the jokes and watch the professional timing; the punch-line comes at just the right moment for maximum impact – not too soon, not too late – followed by a pause to let the laughter subside so that no one will fail to hear the next word. Timing requires practice, not that lectures are full of jokes

Fourth, assessing your own performance is difficult. Your mentor, if he is honest enough and brave enough, will tell you the bad news and the good. He is more likely than others to give an impartial view, but he may have rather high standards himself and high expectations from you. In the R.A.F. I learnt two pieces of advice which I pass on to you: never volunteer for anything and never underestimate your own abilities when talking to a senior officer. They probably apply to research as much as to flying, but the common fault is to have too low an estimate of competence before a lecture and too high an estimate of success afterwards.

A truth is always a compound of two half-truths, and you never reach it because there is something more to say.

Tom Stoppard

8

WRITING

When you come to write about your own research there will be a great temptation to dress it up, to use flowery language, to show off. Don't. During your library search you will have read many published papers. You may have found the information you sought but you will not have read great literature; on the contrary you will have come to realise that many researchers write badly.

To write well we need three gifts: the command of words, the command of syntax, and the command of rhythm. We should also write for a particular reader but there are two kinds or readers: those who already know about your subject and those who don't. Both want to learn from you, both need clarity but when we talk about clarity in research writing we are talking about two separate things: a well thought-out idea (experiment, or conclusions, or the project in general), that is the technical aspect, and good clear writing, that is the language and communication aspect.

Of course, if the technical side is not clear to you it will not be possible to put it in understandable prose but this is rarely the real problem. The problem is much simpler, one of education. It isn't that nurses, doctors, engineers, administrators, scientists and so on can't write: they just prefer to continue a peaceful co-existence with the English language. English, unlike other academic subjects, does not possess a clearly defined teachable body of knowledge; school teachers feel this lack and try to fill the gap with definitions of parts of speech, of phrases and sentences, and with exercises based on them. Language schools for adults do it differently: they concentrate on function. People learn a language to use it and the success of teaching a language has only one criterion – the reaction of the recipient.

In writing we have a choice, but choice operates at different levels. In scientific journals one choice is made for us, indeed imposed on us, by the format in which our prose will be accepted.

What is a good article? "It is one that has a definite structure, makes its point, and then shuts up. Its English uses nouns and verbs and not adjectives and adverbs, while the scientific structure is crisp and each individual section does what it is supposed to and no more".[37] A 50-word prescription that should not be beyond the reach of even a dull fellow. Yet I know tomorrow I will have to read an article which has none of this, and will be hard-going by any standards.

ESSENTIAL TOOLS

You will need the following

Paper and pen.   Use a ball-point pen that you like, that flows freely, and good quality paper so that the physical act of writing is effortless, even sensuous. Goodness knows, the mental effort of placing one word after another is difficult enough, yet the laboriousness of handwriting has a saving grace: it forces the mind to think slowly and deliberately about the use of words because each word costs time and effort to put on paper. Dictation on to a tape recorder tempts us to become rambling, verbose, inexact and slipshod in our use of language. Never use pencil unless you intend to type the final draft yourself.

A good dictionary   for spellings and meanings. A small one on your desk is useful to check spelling – such as the Concise Oxford Dictionary – but the Shorter Oxford Dictionary (in two volumes for preference) is the one to browse through and to consult for unexpected meanings. Use it to find the right word.

Roget's Thesaurus for alternative words or, more importantly, as a stimulus to you to conjure up the apt word. Use it for inspiration as much as for memorable words.

The Complete Plain Words, originally by Sir Ernest Gowers, now revised by Sir Bruce Fraser,[25] is a book to read before you write, to mark those passages that interest you particularly and then refer to them during the stages of writing and revision.

Modern English Usage. Originally written by H.W. Fowler, later revised by Sir Ernest Gowers,[24] is a kind of dictionary of usage with the difference that one is compelled to read on and to follow the various cross-references. Try to become familiar with it before you write, consult it when stuck with a phrase or sentence, but dip in for a quick read whenever you can. There are excellent thumb-nail descriptions of words and their use to help one learn the craft of clear writing.

THE PAPER FOR PUBLICATION

Is it important to be published? Fairfax and Moat[22] answered the question in this way: "If you're a fine cobbler it's your concern to make good shoes. You make them well and that is your satisfaction. They wear well and are comfortable and that is a satisfaction to others, and their satisfaction gives you added satisfaction . . . If you discover a cure for cancer, what is your satisfaction: the discovery or the publication of the discovery, or the fact of seeing people cured? Or all three?" There is another aspect. Without publication, research is sterile. If you have done fine work and made a discovery, it is wrong that you do not pass on the good news and hold it up to criticism.

People often ask, when has the time come to publish? The answer is simple. Publish as soon as you have something worthwhile to report. There is no point in waiting until every loose end has been tied up because that never happens and you could wait for ever: some do! If you develop the research mind there will always be more questions than answers, and the answers you provide will generate questions anyway. This does not mean that you pass on sloppy research, rather that you let others know when you have some evidence to display and are ready to defend it.

There are two things that publication of research will never do. First, it will never prove that you are any good as a researcher. Second it will not even prove that you are a researcher. But it will show that you can do a piece of work, write it up and persuade an editor that it is worth publishing. That alone is an achievement. Value for money in research means results, and results mean publication. So, in spite of what others may say, the best criterion of a successful researcher is still the quality (and usually the quantity) of his publications. If you have no publications to your name, how can you be judged?

Pick your journal with care. Go for the most appropriate to your subject and the most prestigious in your specialty. Then read the "Instructions to Authors" (and they vary greatly between journals: some have none), photocopy them for reference as you write and stick within the "house rules". If you don't, your gem may fail on a technical fault or at best gather unfavourable comment.

In medicine, and similarly in other disciplines, all papers submitted for publication must follow a certain form, the IMRAD structure – Introduction, Material and Methods, Results and Discussion. The author need not adhere rigidly to these headings, indeed many complain that they are unduly restrictive, but they have advantages for writer and reader.[10,18,36] The writer knows what he must include in composing his paper and the reader knows where to find it. In addition, the writer does not have to search for headings to relieve the tedium of a page of prose. How does it all work out in practice? Remarkably well, if you understand what each section implies.

Introduction.   What does this mean? It means just this for the reader: here is the position as I saw it before starting my research project. This is my interpretation of the reading and thinking I have done, the people I have talked to, and what I think needs doing.

Material and Methods.   This is what I used, what I did, how I did it, to whom I did it. It is how I approached the problem, my plan of attack.

Results.   This is what I discovered. The order of discovery and the order of its announcement are rarely the same so tell the important news first. In writing a report full details would be put in an appendix so that you don't swamp the reader with more than he can take in and don't appear too clever: some journals now state that detailed results are available from the author, but not printed in the article.

Discussion.   What inferences do I draw from my work? Do others agree with them (from published papers)? What are the implications? Is my analysis reasonable? What does this mean for the future? Dare I speculate? Should I argue the case for and against my ideas? This is not the place for great advocacy but this section does three things: it draws together your own findings, it relates them to those of others, and it allows you to place both in relation to other knowledge and give some sense of perspective. The rhetoric has to be in keeping with your subject.

Conclusions.   Some of these have become clear in the discussion, as a logical outcome of your work. Often the conclusions will be recommendations.

Acknowledgements.   There should be no fawning, but a straight "thank you" to the grant-giving body, to outsiders who provided material assistance, and to your mentor if he has added to your own ideas.

References.   These are to help the reader rather than to support you. Most journals prefer a certain style (the Vancouver is popular) but you must record the name and initials of the author, the journal or book, date, volume and page numbers accurately. Such detail will be available from your literature-search cards.

Illustrations.   These should be used only to help the reader. So the choice is usually between illustration and typescript? What is the best form? What will the journal accept? Will the illustration reproduce well in that journal?[54,58,59]

Summary or abstract.   This is composed last but may be placed by the editor at the beginning of your paper. A good summary or abstract should, in 150 to 200 words, provide answers to these five questions:-

1. What did you do?
2. Why did you do it?
3. How did you do it?
4. What did you find?
5. What does it mean?

When well written, the abstract sells the research: it extends the title by telling the reader what the paper is about. It provides a reference map because it is a shortened version of the work, it will be read by those who don't want to read much, and can be reproduced as a short report for wide circulation (there are numerous journals devoted entirely to selling abstracts, and for many people these are essential reading in their specialty).

The title.   You had this at the planning stage, before the research started. Now is the time to re-examine it. Is it accurate? Does it indicate what the work is all about? Is it appealing? Can it be shortened? Does it contain the important and essential words for an indexing agency? Can I think of a better title? A good title has four attributes.

1. Correct because it tells you accurately about the subject.
2. Complete in that it limits the amount of information and is therefore precise and not vague.
3. Comprehensible so that everyone in that discipline who would normally read the journal can understand it.
4. Concise because the title expresses the content of the article in the shortest and most efficient way. This inevitably requires you to cut out the deadwood such as "an investigation into . . ., a study of . . .", and so on.

Few titles meet all these criteria: the majority miss on one, some on two, and a few are blatantly misleading. The title you wrote before you started the project will not be worded the same as the title for your published paper: it is the latter which will be indexed in reference books, so get it right.

The person who writes a paper under these ten headings, answering the questions noted in each section, will have a workmanlike report of his research. The act of writing has but one aim: achievement. So how do we go about it.?[5,10,18,26,28,33,36,46,47,49,52]

THE WAY TO WRITE

A lot of people think that writing is an activity in which one scribbles words on paper and then forgets about them. This is probably how you were taught to write a school essay but when there is a need to write, as there is for your research to reach print, one can put on paper roughly what one wants to convey and go back later to consider how best to say it. This is the process known as drafting. Moreover, you can work on the draft until you arrive at a version to be proud of. Even a first draft is often the product of an earlier draft in note form, and the final draft is the best for the journal of your choice. So how many drafts? Opinions vary, but there will be a minimum of four, although some parts of an article will need more, others less, and some will be right first time.

But consider this. Writing is not a one-off affair with little or no development between drafts. Writing improves writing because writing is a skill and, like any other skill, improves with practice and rusts with disuse. You will have the original written protocol of your project, your notebooks, results, and literature-search cards – you already have almost too much. Begin by sorting out what you have already, before adding to it; read and think, then try to turn as much of the data as you have into illustrations – graphs, charts, diagrams, tables. These may be drawn in rough, but not sloppily: there is no point in converting numbers into a diagram that lacks punch.

For the first draft write continuously and quickly from your notes and headings. Try to write a complete text preferably at one sitting so that there is continuity of style. Start writing what interests you most or that which you have at "your finger tips", such as the results of your experiments. Don't worry about good English at this stage. Don't hang about; don't stop to search for missing data, just leave blanks for dates, references, or further points of detail that require looking up. Write fast and leave plenty of room between the lines. When you have finished for the day, either stop in mid-sentence or leave a new heading and notes in preparation for the next day. Time spent wondering what to write when you sit down is valuable time wasted. Try not to read what you have written: you may feel depressed by the deathless prose and not wish to finish. Until you have written a complete first draft, you have nothing to revise, nothing to work at, nothing to show for your research.

Leave the manuscript alone for a few days then read the whole paper for sense and continuity. Mark in the margin those passages that are not clear or that need explanation. The second draft is mostly addition. Add what has been left out, add what needs explaining, add to statements that are not clear. The manuscript is now bigger and probably too long for easy reading.

The third draft has one message: trim it down. Cut out the repetition, the verbiage, and the unnecessary explanations. Each draft should be left to mature: not for years as you would a fine brandy but long enough for you to see your own mistakes when you return to it – the gauche writing, misuse of words, errors of fact, and even sheer dullness. Your paper must attract readers to have any impact. A month is about enough between drafts although not many people can afford that amount of time, or wish to.[47]

In the fourth draft, examine the structural order: move paragraphs around until the whole appears logical and flows. Fit in the illustrations and see how much writing can be omitted thereby. Then examine the English, sentence by sentence. Tinker with the script, adding connecting phrases and sentences as required, but all the time aiming for clarity.[13,16]

Cut-and-stick is a rapid method for rewriting because it allows you to rearrange paragraphs, changing their order without having to write a single word. Cut out the offending paragraph from the page with scissors (clip the remaining loose pieces of paper together so that they are not "lost"), cut through the place where you wish that paragraph to go, apply dry glue stick to the edges and drop it in to make a new page. When you have done this a few times it all looks a mess, but remounting the whole on to a clean blank sheet restores it to a workable document. It makes good sense to delay the final typing until all corrections have been made. Some authors object to adhesives and recommend that inserts should be stapled in place, arguing that the staple is more certain to retain what is required and can be removed easily if you change your mind and wish to move the paragraph elsewhere. My experience is that staples snag on loose sheets and are a nuisance.

The final draft must:

- Be typed, double spacing, with good margins (say 3cm each side).
- Be read and checked for errors of spelling, numerals, or references.
- Always be shown to your mentor for constructive comments.
- Be compared with other articles in the journal of your choice. Count the number of words so that you can compare the size of your article with that of another on a similar topic. Word counting is a good discipline for any author: I am obsessive about it.

When you have written and corrected your final draft, send it with a short covering letter to the journal of your choice. It may be rejected, not because it was bad but more likely because there were several papers of the same quality (quality here means scientific merit and writing). It was borderline for that journal. Occasionally the editor makes an error of judgement, but he is as keen as anyone to sell his journal and attract customers by keeping the contents to a consistently high standard.

Occasionally your paper will be accepted without alteration: it may be very good or you may be very lucky – the right article at the right time. Editors vary: one said, "Surprise me and I'll publish". If the writing is clear and workmanlike you stand a good chance, but articles usually go to assessors first, experts in your field, who may provide helpful and unsolicited comments. Sometimes, of course, you have picked the wrong journal or the journal has too many articles submitted: most "popular" journals reject 80% of offerings.[37] But don't be put off. If your work is good find the journal that will publish, but don't send round dog-eared, coffee-stained sheets: retype and freshen up. If you get regular rejections, consult your mentor.

A LETTER TO A JOURNAL

If you write a letter to a journal with correspondence columns and it is printed, you can add that to the list of publications included in your curriculum vitae.

There are four good reasons for writing.

First, as a commentary on a paper published in that journal, your letter can contribute usefully to the general discussion: additional data can be presented; speculation, refutation, or support can be the aim.

Second, similarly, a letter is used to reply to critics either of the article (particularly if you were the author) or to letters generated by it. This kind of controversy is the lifeblood of most journals with correspondence columns, and the editor often has to exert his authority to stop the flow of lively letters before acrimony creeps in.

Third, as a means of gaining recognition for an original discovery. Researchers like to be "first" and the journal *Nature*, of London, has existed for a century to allow such claims.

Fourth, as a means of publishing negative results. Suppose you plan a neat piece of research, work hard at it, but discover nothing new, only confirming what other people thought (but you hoped to overturn that view which didn't come off), what are you to do with the results? No journal editor is likely to welcome your carefully written, neatly typed, well-documented gem. It has no appeal. There are several ways round the problem. The paper can be "written off" as "experience", hiding your tears of disappointment, or held until such time that you have to give a lecture or write a review of that subject when your own work can be quoted legitimately, but only just, as "Personal Communication (1984)". Or you can write a letter to a journal giving a brief summary of the findings either by joining the ranks of current letter-writers or starting from scratch in the hope that the editor will see it as a likely "hare".

Of course you don't just write to the journal, you write to the editor and your letter is rather formal.

- Open with Sir, or Dear Sir.

- Keep it as short as you can, but include the meat of your research. Count the words of published letters to get some idea of the average maximum length allowed. Brief letters get printed, long letters rejected.

- Quote the names of others who have published in the same field. Give full references at the end of your letter.

- Some journals will accept simple tables or charts, which may get your message over better and quicker, and will improve the appearance of the letter.

- Write in clear, concise English with the minimum of discussion – the other letter writers will do that for you.

- Sign off with your name, qualifications, department and institute with full address in the hope that a like-minded researcher will contact you later.

A TOUCH OF STYLE

What is style? Style is the way you and I write. That's all. If you want to write well and become known by your writing as well as by the quality of your research, that's where style comes in.[10,18,36,61] Let us consider good style under three headings, while admitting that style is quite difficult to define yet easy enough to recognise.

First, elegance and beauty. St Thomas Aquinas wrote in his vast "Summa": "Beauty includes three conditions; integrity or perfection, since things that are imperfect are by that very fact ugly; due proportion or harmony; and lastly brightness and clarity". We need beauty and there is beauty in research, in writing. The dictionary defines style as "those features of literary composition which belong to form and expression rather than to the substance of the thought or matter expressed". So style is giving a solid shape to your communication, and pleasing the reader. In writing we communicate more than we realise because communication is a relationship, and we make a judgement when we read another's writing.

Beauty and elegance start with the design of our research project, continue with the way we tackle it and are permanently recorded in the way we write. Our writing may generate new knowledge, new ideas, and usually new questions to answer, but there can be beauty in those too. Curiously, an elegant experiment tends to beget an elegant result, and elegant results demand stylish prose.

Second, the handling of language. If you can look at a blurred piece of writing and discover clarity merely by making nouns and verbs strong, by cutting out adjectives and adverbs which so often ruin the thing they are supposed to support and make precise, you are editing. If you can cut padding in other ways, to remove the unnecessary, the tautology, the subjective commentary or the trivial opinion, to emphasise the important, you will find that sentences fall into place: they mean what you wish to say. Then remove jargon,[10,20] a vice many flirt with that quickly leads to addiction, and you will begin to develop individual style in writing from the way you organise arguments, arrange units of thought – that is sentences and paragraphs – and make clear what you wish to say by using the appropriate, if not the right words. In choosing words, prefer the familiar to the unfamiliar, the non-technical to the technical, the concrete to the abstract, the plain to the pretentious.

It is easy to believe that complex English is more scientific than ordinary everyday language, but it is a mistake because we all have limited vocabularies: first, the words we easily understand and use frequently, perhaps only 3,000 words; second, words we use for special occasions, another 3,000 at most; third, words we hear or see and think we understand, perhaps another 1,000. Accuracy is not a virtue but a duty in research papers. The accurate word is specific, precise, forceful: find it and use it, but keep it simple. Style uses language effectively and efficiently.

Third, readability. When you have written your masterpiece is there any test to give you some idea how clear it will be to the reader? Yes, there are several.[23,24] The simplest is Robert Gunning's[26] "Fog Index", an indicator of foggy or unclear prose. The Fog Index is calculated by adding the average number of words in the sentences of a representative page of text (A) to the number of three or more syllable words of the same text (L) and multiplying this total by 0.4. The formula is therefore, $F = 0.4 (A + L)$.

Fog Index	*Means*	*Commonly found in*
5	Easy reading	Popular newspapers
7–8	Standard texts	Racy novels
9–11	Fairly difficult	Upmarket newspapers

| 12–15 | Difficult reading | Scientific papers generally |
| 17 and above | Very difficult | University theses |

All tests provide three clear guides in revising your own test. First, use short words and try not to use more than about 150 syllables per 100 words.

Second, use short sentences. Do not exceed 14 words per sentence, and when there are more than 20 words recast that sentence. Third, add human interest by using names, personal pronouns, or words having a gender, when the opportunity arises. The assumption that word length and sentence length determine readability makes it look too simple. There are other factors: good style demands variety and interest, and an answer to the question, "Does it make sense?" As Doris Wheatley said in a radio interview about her job as a professional technical writer: "I write for idiots". Style shows itself in the relationship between form and content: the relationship can harmonise or conflict. In the end, the content has to be acceptable and the form pleasing. Your mentor will help you there but he will not create style for you: that is your responsibility, your privilege.

YOUR MENTOR

If he is good – and he was your choice – he will accept, read and comment on your gem. But note the following five points.

First, he will not rewrite your article for you, even though this may be the easier thing to do, because you have to learn the craft of writing well; it is painful and usually productive, but so is childbirth. A good paper is your child. Occasionally a mentor will be the grammarian who frets about any variation from standard English –

worse than Fowler, who is pretty tolerant – and as a result your racy style is reduced to a dull grey prose. This is much more likely to happen if he attempts to rewrite instead of proposing key ideas of construction which you can slot in or ignore. Do not expect more than a paragraph or two of your mentor's writing, perhaps as an example to follow, because he will be aware that you must establish your style which you recognise and enjoy. By all means discuss, but don't deliberately try to imitate.

Second, he will spell out criticisms, itemise them, be detailed and specific. The terse phrase, "could do better", helps no one.

Third, he should be prepared to justify his stand – hence you are free to argue your own point of view and should do so as a method of learning the skill of clear writing.

Fourth, he will emphasise the major errors and will comment only briefly on spelling or punctuation. He knows that authors are touchy. He will try to be tactful and may not put every criticism down on paper, preferring to talk it over with you. A good mentor will take his pupil through line-by-line but only if the work is savable and correctable. Many are not. The astute mentor will sit and ask and listen and comment. In spoken English the work has clarity, economy, beauty: in written English it has none. So what went wrong? How is it that someone can describe his research in simple, clear, comprehensible language, and then write the same stuff in woolly, confused, unreadable prose? I don't know. It is a complete mystery, but so common that this alone is the best reason for subjecting your writing to an interested and knowledgeable third party.

Fifth, he must be consistent in criticism, and should assume some responsibility if the editor of the journal selected comments adversely, changes the script, or pronounces unfair judgements.

On the other hand:-

● You will only ask your mentor to read and comment on a piece of writing that you consider fit for publication. Never show your mentor a first draft; he must be allowed to judge your literacy on the final draft, for how otherwise can he know how good you really are? Your second best won't do.

● The typescript will be a top copy with only a few corrections and you will hand over a similar photocopy on which he may prefer to work.

● You should realise that you are receiving a favour and that your mentor wants to see your paper in print as much as you do.

● You will have edited your own writing until you think it is right. Every time we change a word, add a phrase or recast a sentence of our own writing we become an editor. But this is rarely enough. We need the eye of a third party for an independent judgement of the quality of our writing. Does it match the quality of the research? If not, we have failed. The expert eye must know his business, your subject, and have good standards himself. Always submit your first three papers to your mentor: you want them to be good so that others will recognise you for your worth. Even when you have enough experience to go it alone you will still need criticism and praise: a mentor will do both. But above all you want your paper published in the right journal: a good mentor will help there too.

Does it not follow that by drilling ourselves to write perspicuously we train our minds to clarify their thoughts?

Sir Arthur Quiller-Couch

9

A THESIS

When your paper has been accepted for publication there follows a long wait. Nothing seems to happen until one day you receive proofs and an order form for reprints which, to your surprise, turn out to be expensive. When the paper is eventually published it all seems rather flat and no one asks you for a reprint for months. What are you to do during this period of waiting? There is a choice. You could abandon research altogether: put it down to experience and hope that it will be useful at some time in the future.

The original research project could be enlarged because there were some loose ends to tie up and the questions raised seem answerable, and perhaps during the project another was born on the way, novel and not related. This phenomenon is well recognised. As you finish one project another begins; indeed you will probably see and think about it before you finish the first. It is easy to develop a "butterfly mind" flitting from one idea to another, and at the end of the day produce nothing of worth. The trouble is that the most exciting part of research is too often the planning of what to do and the dreaming that it will happen: it is addictive and a powerful deterrent to starting real work.

There are of course other reasons for continuing to do research. In the first place, the researcher does not know whether he is any good. In the second place, there is for the research only one proof of identity that is incontrovertible and meaningful: the strange evidence that he continues research. Or you could consider writing a thesis.[10,29,30]

WHY NOW?

Why have a chapter on writing a thesis in a book that is supposed to be for the beginner? Why indeed? I will tell you.

If you have done a little research, had one or two papers accepted for publication, you are still a novice whether you admit it or not. Yet now is the time to consider a thesis seriously. You will need to write a 2,000 word summary of what it will be about, and divide the whole into say fifteen chapters so that the contents of one chapter will follow naturally to the next. The flow and consistency of language and style comes from writing the thesis at one "sitting": polishing comes from revision. This is exactly what the novelist does. Indeed the two occupations have much in common. In both, details of each chapter are largely unknown at an early stage – for the novelist, because he has not developed his characters and the plot – for the researcher, because he has neither devised nor done the necessary experiments. Both have a good idea which has to be worked on. Both need a story line from which to blossom, but we musn't push the simile too far and we have not answered the question: why write a thesis?

If you have had a paper or two published, and without too much trouble, you may begin to wonder if you have the talent to write for the market-place. To the question, are you a writer? there is only one answer: try. Either you can write for popular journals that pay for articles – and if you get paid £70 for 1,000 words you learn to count words as second nature – or you can write for a status symbol, a university thesis, in which case you will have to pay the university for the privilege but it will be a good investment for your career. You may be able to call yourself "doctor" without the need to stick your hands in blood! To a university, a thesis is something else: it is the visible evidence of self-discipline, a certain amount of special education, and usually a minor advance in human knowledge. It is not meant to be the complete answer to a problem, rather the answer to a question posed, an event in a wide spectrum of ignorance. Theses have been written on the subject before yours and theses on the same subject will be written after. In every case the thesis will be judged on four aspects:-

1. Originality and scientific merit of work done personally.
2. The method of examination of an important problem and how it was tackled.
3. Evidence of its educational value for the writer.
4. Conformity of style.

For the university you have to write a book, a book that no publisher in his senses would touch, yet for a small band of intellectuals it is a sacred object. The book is of about 100 to 200 typed pages on A4 paper, bound in a nondescript cover with your name on the spine in gold block – the only evidence of spendthrift luxury – and an edition limited to four copies. Yet the university will treat it like newly-panned gold: if good, retained; if bad, rejected. Like other people the university expects value for money, even if it is your money at stake. And like everyone else the university is concerned to maintain a standard whatever that may mean; standards are difficult to define, are changing all the time and usually imply "the best to date". Hence your own effort may have raised the standard of acceptance for the one who follows you.

The dictionary defines a thesis as a proposition stated, especially when there is a theme to be discussed and proved, or to be maintained against attack. It is related to, but distinct from, the word hypothesis. Since 1653 it has also meant a written dissertation delivered by a candidate for a university degree. In mediaeval universities, and until recently in Sweden, the candidate not only presented his written document to every member entitled to it, but had to defend his thesis by public argument while it was attacked by professors, doctors and graduates of his own university! Such hustings have fallen from fashion; today few universities even require candidates to attend personally for an oral examination on what they have written, which I think is a pity.

BEFORE YOU START TO TAKE IT SERIOUSLY

First think, then get hold of a copy of the university regulations that apply to the thesis you have in mind. Read the small print to make sure that you qualify for admission: if in doubt, write to the university registrar for clarification and if necessary an interview. Better still, talk it over with your mentor and then talk to someone who has presented a successful thesis: take an hour of his time to discover the difficulties and learn about "form", then pop in to look over his thesis – particularly if he fails to show it to you at that consultation – to find out if what he said agrees with what he wrote. You may think you could do better.

If you have to submit the title and a synopsis to the board of studies of the university, before starting to write your thesis, compose these with care and do seek advice. Every word counts. The title must be crisp, clear, unambiguous and interesting.

Now write a 2,000 word outline sketch of what you propose to do, what you hope to find and how you will go about it. Divide this into 15–20 parts, one for each chapter, and you have the skeleton of a thesis. Or have you? What have you got? Something below standard or something beyond your capacity, or is it about right? Seek expert help. Then ask yourself, is it going to be worth it? Don't abrogate personal responsibility for decision-making; don't let others tell you what to do as they will in an academic department – tell them what you are going to do.

Let it be known that you are writing a thesis unless this will irritate influential people.

Proportions are important. If the aim is to end up with a document of 100–150 pages of text then:

Experiments and results ∼ 50% of the total, say 50–75 pages.

Discussion and conclusions ∼ 25% of the total, say 50–75 pages.

Materials and methods
(unless these are original) ∼ 10% of the total, say 10–20 pages

Introduction and proposal ∼ 15% of the total, say 15–25 pages.

There is a guide[44] for consulting other theses, the successful ones: Aslib's "Index to Theses Accepted for Higher Degrees by the Universities of Great Britain and Ireland and the Council for National Academic Awards" will be found in a university library, but it is not easy to read another person's thesis. It is simpler to glance at a few representative theses in the library of your institute, to note the general format, because past pupils have a habit of donating a copy to their alma mater as proof of erudition and accomplishment. The more perceptive people realise that many theses have nowhere else to go and might as well collect dust undisturbed and preserved in a friendly house as take a chance in strange surroundings. It is sad that so few are consulted by freshmen later, but heartening to realise that the new will not follow too faithfully the old.

STRUCTURE AND ORGANISATION

The structure is conventional, with minor variations between different theses and different universities, and hence organisation can be based on these.

Title   for a thesis should be pithy and informative and, as with any paper for publication, is rarely the one you started with. Indeed, for a thesis there are always at least two titles: the first sets out to define and confine the problem and is temporary, the second is the final, short, permanent, and apt title.

The first title should be descriptive: it will be the "pole star" to which the work is directed. It defines the problem you are going to write about, because the precise definition of a problem enables you to concentrate on what really matters and provides a clear aim, it prevents you wasting time on irrelevancies, helps you to be clear about what you are trying to do and may provide a direct clue to the most successful course of action, and makes it easier to explain to others what you are trying to do.

Preface   is a short statement of about 50 words in which the author states the object of the work, why it was done, the methods used, what hypothesis was tested and what was found. It can usefully be combined with the *summary* to form a synopsis, to substitute for both.

Acknowledgements   may be placed next, or at the end. This is usually a list of all those who helped in any way and it must be complete to avoid offending anyone: it is often a source of surprise, and sometimes embarrassment, to your supervisor. Acknowledge all facilities made available, research grants, equipment, drugs, the typist, but limit the eulogy to one page.

Summary   or synopsis. This describes the contents of the thesis in 200–250 words and is the piece that the assessor reads first to discover what has been done, why, and what has been found. If he remains confused after reading, and does not understand, he will be reluctant to read the rest with any enthusiasm. The summary can be modelled on that given in the previous chapter on writing a paper for publication.

Survey of previous work or historical review   In order to understand one's own times and work it is necessary to have an historical perspective. It is impossible to look at an object or view without being aware of the existence of perspective, the optical effect which gives a sense of distance and three-dimensional solidity to what is seen. It is equally impossible for the researcher to work without a sound knowledge of the general perspective of what has gone before in his subject. If this perspective is distorted the subsequent research is likely to follow the same distortion.

What is relevant to the architect may also be of value to the researcher. Parallel railway lines appear to come together as they recede into the distance; this is known as "convergence" and similarly our ideas converge as we look back. The spaces between telegraph poles appear to get smaller as they recede from the spectator even though we know that they are equally spaced: this is known as "foreshortening". The telegraph poles appear to become smaller as they recede from the spectator: this is known as "diminution". There are two other features: detail of objects, and their tone and colour, diminish with distance.

We can think of the history of the subject for the thesis as a row of events, like telegraph poles, which stretch into the distant past. We can provide dates and list the events in correct order. But this is not what is meant by an historical review. It fails to give the perspective view. It is not history either. Hugh Trevor-Roper, Professor of Modern History at Oxford, defined the word at his valedictory address in 1980: "History is not how things were, but how things were in relation to what they might have been". This does not mean that a library search becomes a minor feature for thesis construction, rather the reverse: copious notes from wide reading, time to think deeply, and much discussion, particularly with your tutor, are more important than ever. The purpose of recalling the past is to educate the present, or at least to discover what went wrong. In this context it is often valuable to read editorials (usually in general journals) for current views of the subject at the time the papers being consulted were written: the unanswered questions are commonly spelt out, and sometimes with useful speculation.

But at the end you have to be able to make a statement, "this is my interpretation of the past". The next statement, "this is the problem as I see it", relates directly to the one before and the sequence must be logical. The third statement, "and this is how I propose to solve the problem, or more correctly to answer the question posed" is related again to what has gone before and to your personal interpretation of history. So you see, the section on the historical survey is an important part of the thesis: and, in my experience, the most difficult to do well. It is all too easy to write 100 pages of history copied from books, yet miss the point of what has been read. The survey must not take up more than a quarter of the total space: the thesis is about your work, your results, not what others did. As the artist uses perspective, to see more detail of an object viewed from a short distance, so too the thesis must give detail of your research and omit that of others. Perspective is what is seen from a fairly specific viewpoint: it does not automatically exclude any other viewpoint. Perspective, for the artist, is the most accurate system yet evolved to produce as nearly as possible, the drawing of a three-dimensional object which coincides with the actual view of the object seen from the chosen viewpoint. The artist chooses his place to stand, and so too does the thesis writer but he must believe passionately in his stance, to carry conviction in his perspective.

It may be impossible to avoid a certain simplification,

but the reasons for so doing should be set out. You may justifiably wish to emphasise some features which have influenced the direction of your own work. You should begin the survey at the appropriate stage of development of your subject and not willy-nilly.

Good advice is to pose a list of say six questions derived from your interpretation of reading the literature. You know you are going to answer these questions – they constitute the main body of the thesis – but it makes the whole thing more interesting for the assessors who have to read your gem: it focuses the minds of author and assessor on the real problems.

Materials and methods may cover several chapters. New techniques will need to be validated, the methods of statistical analysis described and the reliability of methods of assessment recorded. The population from which the test sample was taken must be described in detail. This section is important. One of the assessors may well have an international reputation in the technical methods you use, and will be critical of any errors.

Results can be reported fairly briefly. Many will be as tables, charts and graphs: their design and artistic appearance help to lift the thesis above the ordinary. As Hawkins[29] so rightly pointed out: "Although only relevant results and successful experiments need be described in detail, unsuccessful experiments and the wrong turnings which are inevitable in all research should be recorded". These "wrong turnings" sometimes turn out useful later, either to yourself or to another. It is wise to omit comment on the results, or at least severely limit it, until the next section on discussion.

Discussion starts a new chapter. This is the place to comment on the results, interpret them, and draw appropriate deductions without recapitulation of the results. The conclusions lead on naturally and tend to fall into three parts:

1. The conclusions derived from your own work.
2. The relationships of your work to that of others.
3. Speculation on where the conclusions might lead.

Up to now you should have kept apart, scrupulously, fact from fiction and never mixed the two: this is the place to mix them to produce what T.V. calls "faction", but make clear what you are discussing.

I suggested that you should pose questions, that you intend to answer, at the end of the literature survey as one method for drawing attention to the main theme of the thesis. If you did so, now is the time to pose new questions brought to light by your own work. In this way it becomes possible to put your thesis in perspective – one brick in the wall of knowledge, and not the entire wall – and so disclose your own maturity and humility. It is also a recognised art form: you started with questions which you answered and at the end you presented new questions for someone else to answer.

References   are always required: a bibliography, that is a complete list of works published on the subject, may be attempted and in some ways is as hard to compose as any chapter. But here are two warnings. First, all references must be accurate, set out according to a recognised method (either Harvard or Vancouver style) which the university may prescribe, and be complete. Assessors have a habit of examining references with particular care and will carry out spot-checks by reading some. The list of references must include all the important relevant publications: any omission will soon be noticed, particularly if an assessor is the author. Second, never ever include publications that you have not read: assessors have the knack of asking for detail about them and giving the impression that the whole thesis is suspect.

References will have been collected on cards, sorted alphabetically before making the list, and tagged to prevent disorder. Because there will be personal notes on the back of each, it has always seemed to me a good idea for the candidate to bring them to the oral examination, as an aide-memoire, although I have never seen anyone do so.

Appendices contain all material which slows down or interrupts unnecessarily the easy reading of the text, such as tables, detailed diagrams, charts and graphs, but any illustration necessary for understanding the text must be placed in the main text. It is not a "junk shop" but an integral part of the thesis where extra detail or extra information can be found if the reader wishes to pursue an item in more depth. Each appendix must be numbered separately and indicated at the relevant point in the text.

THE MECHANICS OF WRITING

Before writing, re-read the university regulations concerning your thesis. Do you still qualify? Is your project sufficient? Is it too difficult to complete in the time available, or at all? These questions will have been asked before: they need to be asked again because it is unwise to leave the writing of the thesis until the end of the research work. The trick is to do most of the writing and reading before you start. That sounds surprising, but it makes sense. You know what you intend to do, so why not write that down (material and methods and some of the discussion); you will have read a fair amount so why not an outline of the historical survey and the hypothesis to be tested? All this will be in note form, but some will be good quality paragraphs which can be slotted in at the appropriate places when serious writing begins.

Importantly, the more you have written early on the more selective you become in your subsequent reading;

the more evident the gaps in your arguments, the more specific and precise your experiments will be to fill them. So there are great advantages in starting to write as soon as you see the way ahead. The main disadvantage is that there may be much to discard later and time appears to have been wasted, but it never is. The technique of writing differs little from that described in the previous chapter, but there are some important differences.

First, collect all your data and spread it all out on a large table, your thesis desk. With notes, tables, and illustrations, and the outline plan you are ready to begin. Decide on longhand or type? Here is the ideal chance to learn to type[56] and the opportunity for plenty of practice with a purpose – your thesis.

Second, it takes just 50 days to write an average length thesis for a PhD or an MD or an MS or even an MA. That is all the time needed for the first draft. You are going to write four pages of longhand or two typed pages every day, seven days a week, for the next 50 days. How? By choosing a quiet place, away from T.V. and other distractions. There are no holidays for thesis writers; there is no time either, so the first requirement is to make time, find time, and the daily stint may be two hours or more; your choice is morning or evening, either get up earlier or go to bed later. Write continuously: keep going, don't dawdle, and if there is a date you can't remember or an idea you want to insert but can't, then leave a space and press on. Dialogue, the life blood of a novel, is not allowed in a thesis but you can talk to yourself and make brief notes in the margin of your writing as reminders of detail to be included or of points to debate.

If you do your own typing, use the cheapest paper for the first draft (and second and third), pencil the page numbers, put the chapter title at the top of each sheet, and never throw anything away: if your writing is wrong, leave four lines and start again. Keep every sentence, every paragraph, in case they are needed later, but they rarely are: "murder your darlings" is the usual order. If writing in longhand, use a ballpoint pen that you like and paper which is easy to write on. Flimsy paper is not the best and always have a thick pad on a firm ground so that your writing is legible and effortless.

Third, start with the easiest part to write. You can, of course, begin at the beginning and work your way straight through but you may regret it: the thrill of seeing the written pages pile up encourages most people to keep going. You know what your thesis is about, you know what each chapter has to do to advance the story, so follow the outline plan and write one sentence at a time and don't worry about the task of writing a whole thesis. Write now, revise later. Read back occasionally, but never revise at this stage: that is a pleasure to come, so reserve it for the time when you have earned it. If you attempt to edit now you will have that job to do all over again later, and that really is inefficient. Don't stop to admire your own writing and never show the first draft to anyone: the prose you have created will be commented on adversely and depress you.

Fourth, pay particular attention to grammar, words, spelling and flow.[13,16,18,20,24,25,46,48,49] The paper for publication will pass through the hands of an editor before it is printed in the journal, your thesis will not. The journal editor will improve your piece, the thesis assessor will not and may demand corrections which are expensive and irritating but must be done to be accepted. Forget about style at this stage: it will evolve with drafting, but do look at sentences and make each do one thing only for you; chop up long sentences into smaller, but keep variety of length for rhythm and interest. Check spelling: errors tend to be perpetuated until you become blind to them. Ask yourself where additional material fits best? Should there be an extra chapter, or a new heading elsewhere? Try to get some idea of balance at this stage by keeping chapters about the same length. Juggle with rearrangement of the order of things until you achieve a logical and pleasing flow. The freedom of composition inherent in writing a thesis should be enjoyed and used to the author's advantage. This freedom, not normally accorded to the research writer but natural to the novelist, is often neglected and as a result many theses are full of stuffy prose as though produced to a formula, when they could be so much more exciting for the reader. Decide how to break the monotony of a whole page of type. How should paragraphing be done? Where do illustrations, examples, and quotations fit? How will they be referred to? Avoid duplication and repetition – illustrations or text, not both. Finally, start on the English language. Remove most adjectives, adverbs, "very", "it", and clichés. Examine words: consult the dictionary for meaning and the "Thesaurus" for alternatives. Use commonsense, but keep tinkering with your piece: worry at it, until satisfied.

Fifth, get ready for the final draft. Start by reading the whole. Does it make an interesting story? Can you change the order of the writing to improve the logic of the argument? Is there unity in the flow of writing? Are there errors of fact, of logic, or of reasoning? At this stage it is not a thesis but a mess of paper, fortunately still in correct order but some pages are shorter or longer than others and the whole is becoming unworkable. Now is the time to retype some pages leaving ample margins for further corrections. Do a quick check for "readability".

Examine each sentence again. Does it do what you want it to do? Is the sentence effective? Is it still too long? Cut out "clever" sentences, vague words and jargon. Revise paragraph by paragraph, page by page, trimming and editing until the whole is finely tuned. Polished writing requires elbow grease and a hard heart. Finally, revise the title to make it crisper and more appropriate to the work you have actually done: the final title may be quite different from the one you started with.

The manuscript now looks worse than ever. Now read

from start to finish, swiftly, making minor repairs only. You'll be surprised, I hope, at what you have accomplished. You may think it "the greatest thesis ever" or that "it drags in spots". Tinker away a little more until satisifed. It will never be absolutely right and probably one could continue to review and re-write for ever but that is not the idea. When you have been through four or five drafts, making worthwhile changes each time, then you have done your best. Now stop – stop cold. The thesis is finished.

THE FINAL COPY

This is the typescript which will be submitted as a bound volume to the university. If four copies are required you can submit a top and three carbon-copies or you can make photocopies. Most universities have regulations on the exact nature of binding and will supply a list of approved binders.

● Have the final copy typed by a professional. You will have to pay but if you have done good work, written a good script, it is money well spent. Use standard typeface, pica or élite, and never fancy script or imitative cursive.

● Use good quality bond paper and buy enough for the whole thesis: minor variations in paper size – almost always A4 (297 × 210 mm) – do occur and spoil the appearance of the final bound volume.

● Always have enough prints made of the illustrations so that you can furnish each volume. If you use special thin and flexible printing paper the illustrations can be integrated into the text and the legends for each typed below on that paper to give a sense of unity. Airmail-weight photographic paper of all grades of contrast used to be available. Now we have only Kodak P84 Grade 2 (average, or standard contrast) for photographs, but for line-work there are varieties of document-copying paper available as A4 size sheets. Line-work such as graphs and charts, always looks better on high contrast paper. The messy business of mounting photographs on plain sheets, which always buckle, the risk of them falling out, and the distressing appearance of an overstuffed album are all neatly avoided. For the assessor who has to read your thesis, the ideal offering is "thin and crisp and even" which applies to the appearance as much as to the writing.

- Give precise written instructions to the typist: double spacing always; type on one side of the paper only; prescribe the margins – 4cm on left, for binding, and 2cm on the right, with 2.5cm top and bottom – or as directed by the university regulations, which are usually specific for the binding (and often there is an official list of recognised bookbinders).

- All pages must be numbered and it is usually easier to do this with an automatic stamper after binding, but the "contents" pages must carry the correct numbers.

- Every page typed must be read for errors of typing. Now is not the time to rewrite your script, but if a page needs retyping it is justifiable to alter the text – and it may cost money. In general, tinkering at this stage is rarely worthwhile; the tension is too great, the urgency to dispatch to the university too obvious, and having lived with it for so long there is little originality to insert. So leave it alone.

- Always keep a copy of everything to do with your thesis: put a copy of the bound volume in the bank in case of fire, floods, earthquake, theft, total loss.

- Place bound copies in cardboard boxes to protect the binding and corners – two at a time or all four together – because the postman may not realise the value of that heavy package. If the university office is nearby, deliver by hand; if not, post to the correct address and enclose a stamped-addressed postcard for acknowledgement. ("Thesis received, four copies", and a space for signature and date). This is a polite gesture even though the university will usually write you a note. Some universities have delivery dates to be met because theses may be considered only twice yearly.

● Sit back and relax; you may not have finished with the thesis yet but you can begin to think of other things. Usually within 2–4 months you will hear from the university: the date for an oral examination, pass, fail, or revise and resubmit.

● For the oral examination, read through your thesis a week before, bring a copy with you, and attend with confidence.

When it is all over you will have to present the top copy to the university library, place one in the library of your own institution, and offer a copy to your supervisor who may wisely and kindly decline. Keep a copy, your very own, nearby to handle and relive those industrious days: but never try to get it published as a book because it was never intended to be one.

MENTOR OR SUPERVISOR?

When you decide to continue research and write a thesis you will, of course, tell your mentor. He in turn may indicate those areas where you need further tuition – the lack of concentration, the butterfly mind, the need to write and speak better – hardly encouraging, but well meant. When you talk over with your mentor the decision to present a thesis for a higher degree, you will see a subtle change come about. Your mentor will become possessive of you, and relish the intellectual challenge of the university. More than likely he will delight in the chance to teach you from experience because this is his opportunity for true creativity.

Your mentor will change perceptibly to a supervisor, a term curiously absent in many university regulations, but without supervision the production of a thesis is harder than it need be. Your mentor will now point the targets for your research, set the pace, carry out spot checks for quality control and to detect any deviations from the goal. He will "call the shots", make the appointments and you will need to parade with all data at the time stated. Things may take on an air of unwelcomed discipline, of a mini-examination, when you find that suddenly you have a critical editor directing your work.

Do not despair. In due course you will acknowledge, in the thesis, the help you received from your supervisor. This written note, however graciously recorded, will be locked away in the maximum-security section of the university library for all to see yet none consult. Your mentor knows all this but is prepared to trade that honour for the onerous job of becoming your active supervisor NOW. So be grateful, and listen. Your supervisor will obtain his own reward as personal satisfaction of a job well done – your success – and derive little from the eulogy you wrote.

Your supervisor will insist on the thesis outline, help you divide this into the appropriate chapters, check that you have enough data to support the conclusions that you make, that predications can be verified, that arguments and data are presented logically, in the most appropriate form and to best advantage, that expert statistical advice on the sample size and methods of analysis have been obtained beforehand and incorporated into the text later.

Of course, you can do all this on your own, but think of the sweat. The work must be your own and fairly original, but only a fool would refuse a helping hand.

Take one idea, that's plagiarism;
Steal the lot, that's research.
                                    Common Knowledge

10

THE SUMMING UP

There are some things that will never change, such as the fundamental creative process by which a certain number of individuals in every society elect to distil images from their surroundings and construct them into an hypothesis for the education and progress of the rest. These are the researchers, and this book sets out to explain *some* of the methods by which they do so. I am deeply conscious that there is still a great deal left unsaid; that some of the things I have written will be criticised by my colleagues, who have evolved their own systems and view research in a different light. There is no single way to do research, but this book tries to point the beginner in the right direction. By now, if you have completed a project, you are no longer an ignorant novice even though you may still have a lot to learn, as we all have, but you have come to the point where a conscious decision must be made. You have to ask yourself: has it been worthwhile? Will it be useful in my job? Did I enjoy it? If the answer is "yes" to all three questions then, probably, you must continue in research.

The way a researcher sees his role, and the role of those he hopes to work with, is important because it affects his attitude to his own work. It is of vital importance for the future of research in all its many branches that the researcher shall retain his independence of spirit, entering research as a free man who owes nothing to anyone but himself and his subject. Without that determination, the creative process, however fertile in the beginning, will eventually wilt and die. This independence of mind is recognised in scientific merit, is central to it, and it is upon this quality alone that your work will be judged by others.

One quality that really is useful in research – a steely

determination to succeed – is no different from that needed in any other competitive activity. Research is competitive, for ideas, for money, for space, for publications and much more; have no doubts about that. And why not? Research must be seen to be productive and profitable, because it is no longer a luxury but a necessity in all walks of life. It is impossible to plan structured exercises for would-be researchers – as one can in other disciplines such as mathematics or writing – because they would be research projects in their own right. You can of course look around you and identify a problem, then think how to solve it, but you'll never know whether you solved it until you get down to the job and find that the real thing is more exacting and more exciting than any imagination.

New researchers who have had the fortitude to read this book from start to finish will, I hope, avoid wasting much time and many mistakes as they start an exciting occupation. May I sum up the main points that I think are worth drawing to your attention, points that are intended to guide and keep the researcher out of trouble and on the way to success. For convenience I have numbered them to correspond with the chapters of this book.

1. Do consider exposing yourself to research as a form of education which may pay off handsomely in your career. If you have a project that you wish to investigate then take time to think it through, to get it right, and then do it. Research means thinking for yourself.

2. Ideas are the creative side of any job; they make work interesting, bring personal enjoyment, and sometimes company profit. But ideas have to be put into language, communicated to others, and be seen to be practical possibilities. The preliminary tests in chapter two are easily applied before the final test of scientific method. Research is having an idea and the means to test it.

3. Planning can be an end in itself, but if an idea is worthy of the effort of research it is also worthy of a good clean plan from a tidy mind. The ability to plan and

execute are qualities of importance in everyone's life. Research is an orderly process. Research is a plan in action.

4. Reading is something we were taught at school and by puberty no one bothered to teach us more. Yet a book is the most portable, durable, discussable, transportable and clarified form of knowledge that we have. In a lifetime, one can read more than 1,200 books (say 20 each year) or more. But to what purpose? In research, the purpose of reading is clear cut: information pertinent to the current project, or stimulation for future projects. We have to record the essentials of what we read because we are going to use them, so we need a method of recall too. We record our own data for evidence, for publication, for stimulation to others. Research means reading and recording. Chapter four shows you one reliable method of how to do both.

5. Research needs all forms of communication and one of the most valuable, yet permanent, is illustration. Indeed illustration has special advantages because it can transmit more information, more completely and faster than any other method, but with one proviso: the recipient and the transmitter must recognise the message and be quite familiar with the technique. To be at cross-purposes is not to slow down the speed of communication but to destroy it completely. Hence illustrations which replace text in writing or speech in lecturing, must be clear, concise, accurate and comprehensible. Research is a way of illustrating life.

6. In this chapter we consider grants, not the lifeblood of research as many seem to believe, but a means of support without which things would not get done or only slowly. A grant is an investment, not charity, an investment in an idea and a person to put it into practice. Grant-giving bodies take risks (on your promises) and they try to reduce them by requiring factual information. Here we consider some of the ways of applying for money, how to make a realistic assessment of the needs, and how

to report your work. Research costs money.

6A. This is the missing chapter, as you might have guessed, on doing research. When it comes to action you are on your own: front-line in war, or committee debate in peace, it's a lonely job; personal problems have to be suppressed in favour of doing the job you have to do. In the end, no one can help you do it: they can and will advise you, provide a helping hand, but only you can carry out the work that uncovers the evidence to support your idea. And why not? You intend to take the credit. Research is doing your own thing for your own reasons.

7. Having done the work you will seek approval for your actions: don't crow, ask. The best way to ask is to give a lecture on your project. Humility receives its reward in this world in the form you most desire: respect and recognition. To lecture well is an art worth acquiring because speaking is a universal form of communication and probably the most effective: words and gestures can appeal to the heart and mind as no other form of communication can. So, to acquire a good lecture technique is to acquire a valuable skill for use in research. Research is telling others about it.

8. This chapter deals with writing, not just writing about your research project but about the skill of using language to the greatest effect. In research, the written word is the only building block of knowledge which is accepted universally as an advance. Research is preserved by publication.

9. One of the accolades of successful research is the ability to present successfully a thesis to your university. The decision to acquire the status of degree by thesis is best taken early on and this chapter sets out the way to go about it. The demands of universities differ but the aim never changes: the best you can do is the best you will submit for inspection. The technique of organising and writing your thesis is described in detail. Theses are the milestones in research, not the signposts.

In this summing up I have tried to bring all the strands together, hoping that they will make a coherent and helpful pattern. The subject of inspiration is the source of much misunderstanding among those who are not creative themselves; they seek an explanation of the baffling phenomenon which enables man to start research at all. Painting we can understand, nor is there anything esoteric about the concept of literature since, however exalted, it deals with words, the everyday currency of communication. But to discover a problem and solve it, which is what research is all about, is difficult to understand until you have tried. The first requirement of a researcher is to think, the second to ask a question, the third to formulate a possible answer, and the fourth to put it to the test.

There is a myth that researchers work only when "inspired", but in fact they work after careful thought and thorough planning, and as they work there is a certain lubrication and the pace quickens. The inspiration, it is true, comes from out-of-the-blue as it were, but the stimulus is undoubtedly observation, contemplation, reading and doing. The contemplation may occur while doing the washing up or the ironing, painting a door or clearing a gutter: you don't have to assume Rodin's pose, but you do have to use your head.

Research and invention have a lot in common. The inventor sees a need, turns it into a demand, and tries to meet it in a practical and profitable form. The researcher sees a need, turns it into a question which he tries to answer, tells everyone about it, and hopes that he will be remembered for his contribution. Both continue to change their final product, to make it better to find a wider application, and both stand or fall by public opinion: for the inventor this is the purchasing public, the researcher his peers. And in both cases, large numbers of people neither know nor care.

There is great pleasure to be gained from doing good research. It is a means of unique communication with others in one's own and other countries. It is a privilege that should never be abused. People will talk of your work, a just reward, and you will become known (a somebody, never a nobody) and acclaimed or disowned – don't take either to heart – but, I hope, you will remain true to the humble origins of scientific method: evidence above all else.

I do not know whether a majority of my fellow researchers will agree with me, but I feel strongly that every researcher has an opportunity in his publications, by his example too, of strengthening the courage and confidence of his countrymen and of those where original research is frowned on or suppressed. It is still a wonder to me to observe the effect that research can have on the general morale of an institution: people walk tall and are proud of another's reputation. Of course there is one element that is as important to the researcher as it is to the courtroom lawyer or the racetrack punter: luck. Without it the rewards will be slow in coming; with it, Arcadia. I wish you a large slice of luck to go with your hard work.

REFERENCES TO FURTHER READING

What follows isn't an exhaustive bibliography but a brief list of books which you perhaps should read before or in the course of doing your research. Either they demonstrate in practice how research should be done or have something useful to say about research in general. I don't mean that you don't need any others; any book that you read and enjoy has something to teach you, if only about yourself.

There is no publication on this list which I have not read with profit, or which I shall not read again with the pleasure of a different viewpoint. There are not many books which give you original ideas like the selection on the shelf in a supermarket. You have to formulate your ideas from the stimuli that reading about your own and allied subjects, about the world in general, from talking to people, listening to lectures, even dreaming, all provide when those stimuli can reach an open mind. Even when you have an idea, the connection with previous experience or events may not be obvious.

Reading is so important in research that you will have to pick and choose according to your own taste, but publications on method and organisation should always be read. This book does not attempt systematic coverage of all forms of research and it is essentially arbitrary in its selection of topics and in its connection of thought. You can fill in the big gaps it has left and encounter some views different from mine in the list of books and papers that follow. Some books have an asterisk against them; these I recommend that you buy – not all at once but one-at-a-time, and when you have read one buy another – because you will need to refer to them often. None is expensive, all are I think value for money, but the value of having a volume to dip into at will and find what you want cannot be measured in terms of money; convenience is often the greater need.

REFERENCES

1. Balfour M. (1979). *Propaganda in War*, Routledge and Kegan Paul, London.
2. Beck S.D. (1962). *The Simplicity of Science*, Penguin, Harmondsworth.
3.*Beveridge W.I.B. (1980). *Seeds of Discovery*, Heinemann Educational Books, London.
4a. Booth J.D.L. editor (1973). *Directory of Grant-making Trusts*, 3rd compilation, Charities Aid Fund of National Council of Social Services, Tonbridge.
4b. Villemor A. (1983). *Directory of Grant-making Trusts*, 8th compilation, Charities Aid Foundation, Tonbridge.
5. Booth V. (1978). *Writing a Scientific Paper*, 4th edition. Biochemical Society, London.
6. B.M.A. Planning Unit (1976). *Research Funds Guide*, 3rd edition, British Medical Association, London.
7. Bronowski J. (1960). *The Commonsense of Science*, Heinemann Educational Books, London.
8. Bronowski J. (1964). *Science and Human Values*, Penguin, Harmondsworth.
9. Buzan A. (1974). *Use Your Head*, BBC Publications, London.
10.*Calnan J. (1976). *One Way to do Research: The A—Z for those Who Must*, William Heineman Medical Books, London.
11.*Calnan J. and Barabas A. (1981). *Speaking at Medical Meetings: A Practical Guide*, 2nd Edition, William Heinemann Medical Books, London.
12. Calnan J. and Monks B. (1975). *How to Speak and Write: A Practical Guide for Nurses*, William Heinemann Medical Books, London.

13. Carey C.V. (1960). *Mind the Stop*, Cambridge University Press, London.

14. Cooper B.M. (1964). *Writing Technical Reports*, Penguin, Harmondsworth.

15. De Leeuw M. and De Leeuw E. (1965). *Read Better, Read Faster*, Penguin, Harmondsworth.

16. Dirckx J.H. (1976). *The Language of Medicine*, Harper and Row, London.

17. Dover K. (1980). *The Greeks*, BBC Publications, London.

18. Dudley H. (1977). *The Presentation of Original Work in Medicine and Biology*, Churchill Livingstone, Edinburgh.

19. Edinburgh H.R.H. Duke of (1982). *A Question of Balance*, Michael Russell, Salisbury.

20. Elder J.D. (1954). Jargon – good and bad, *Science*; **119**: 536–8.

21. Evans M. (1979). How to use slides. In *How To Do It* (Lock S., ed.). British Medical Association, London.

22. Fairfax J. and Moat J. (1981). *The Way to Write*, Elm Tree Books, London.

23. Flesch R. (1962). *The Art of Readable Writing*, Collyer Macmillan, New York.

24.*Fowler H.W. (1965). *Dictionary of Modern English Usage*, 2nd Edition revised by Sir Ernest Gowers, Oxford University Press, London.

25.*Gowers E. (1973). *The Complete Plain Words*, 2nd Edition revised and added to by Sir Bruce Fraser, H.M. Stationery Office, London.

26. Gunning R. (1952). *The Technique of Clear Writing*, McGraw Hill, New York.

27. Hawkins C.F. (1964). Speaking at Meetings, *Lancet*; **1**: 261–3.

28. Hawkins C. (1967). *Speaking and Writing in Medicine*, Thomas, Springfield.

29. Hawkins C. (1976). Writing the MD thesis, *British Medical Journal*; **2**: 1121–4.

30. Hawkins C. (1979). How to write the MD thesis. In *How To Do It* (Lock S., ed.). British Medical Association, London.

31.*Hill A.B. (1977). *A Short Textbook of Medical Statistics*. The English Language Book Society and Hodder and Stoughton, London.

32.*Huff D. (1954). *How to Lie with Statistics*, Penguin, Harmondsworth.

33. Kirkman J. (1980). *Good Style for Scientific and Engineering Writing*, Pitman, London.

34. Ley P. (1977). Psychological studies of doctor–patient communication. In *Contributions to Medical Psychology* (Rachman S., ed.). Pergamon Press, Oxford.

35. Lional N.D.W. and Herxheimer A. (1970). Assessing reports of therapeutic trials, *British Medical Journal*; 2: 637–40.

36.*Lock S. (1977). *Thorne's Better Medical Writing*, 2nd Edition, Pitman Medical, Tonbridge Wells.

37. Lock S. (1979). How to survive as an editor. In *How To Do It* (Lock S., ed.). British Medical Association, London.

38.*Lock S. editor. (1979). *How To Do It*, British Medical Association, London.

39.*Magee B. (1973). *Popper*, Fontana – Collins, Glasgow.

40. Medawar P.B. (1969). *The Art of the Soluble*, Penguin, Harmondsworth.

41.*Medawar P.B. (1981). *Advice to a Young Scientist*, Pan Books, London.

42. Mitchell J.D. (1964). *How to Write Reports*, Fontana, London.

43. Morton L.T. (1977). *The Use of Medical Literature*, Butterworth, London.

44.*Morton L.T. (1979). *How to Use a Medical Library*, 6th Edition, William Heinemann Medical Books, London.

45. Morton R. (1969), The lantern slide. *Photographic Journal*; **108**: 82–92.
46. O'Connor M. and Woodford F.P. (1978). *Writing Scientific Papers in English: An ELSE—Ciba Foundation Guide for Authors*, Pitman Medical, Tunbridge Wells.
47. Paton A. (1979). How to write a paper. In *How To Do It* (Lock S., ed.). British Medical Association, London.
48. Pei M. (1970). *Words in sheep's clothing (How people manipulate opinion by distorting word meanings)*. Allen and Unwin, London.
49. Pickering G. (1961). Language, the lost tool of learning in Medicine and science. *Lancet*; **3**: 116–19.
50. Popper K. (1972). *Conjectures and Refutations: The Growth of Scientific Knowledge*, 4th Edition. Routledge and Kegan Paul, London.
51. Powell L.S. (1980). *A Guide to the Use of Visual Aids*, 3rd Edition, British Association for Commercial and Industrial Education, London.
52. Rathbone R.R. (1972). *Communicating Technical Information*, Addison-Wesley, Massachusetts.
53. Reichman W.J. (1970). *Use and Abuse of Statistics*, Penguin, Harmondsworth.
54. *Reynolds L. and Simmonds D. (1981). *Presentation of Data in Science: Principles and Practices for Authors and Teachers*, Nijhoff, London.
55. Rose G. and Barker D.J.P. (1979). *Epidemiology for the Uninitiated*, British Medical Association, London.
56. Rowe B. (1981). *Type it Yourself*, Penguin, Harmondsworth.
57. Sandoe E. and Andersen J.D. (1978). *A Guide to Better Slides*, Presented free by Boehringer Ingelheim Ltd.
58. Simmonds D. (1976). The chartist's dilemma. *Medical and Biological Illustration*; **26**: 153–8.

59. *Simmonds D. editor (1980). *Charts and Graphs*, Guidelines for the visual presentation of statistical data in the life sciences. Institute of Medical and Biological Illustration. MTP Press, Lancaster.

60. Stone K. (1966). *Evidence in Science: A Simple Account of the Principles of Science for Students of Medicine and Biology*, Wright, Bristol.

61. Strunk W. and White E.B. (1979). *The Elements of Style*, 3rd Edition, Macmillan, London.

62. *Swinscow T.D.V. (1981). *Statistics at Square One*, 7th Edition, British Medical Association, London.

63. Thring M.W. and Laithwaite E.R. (1977). *How to Invent*, Macmillan, London.

64. Timbury M.C. (1979). How to use the library. In *How To Do It* (Lock S., ed.). British Medical Association, London.

65. Waddington C.H. (1948). *The Scientific Attitude*, 2nd Edition, Penguin, Harmondsworth.

66. Warren M.D. (1979). Plan a research project. In *How To Do It* (Lock S., ed.). British Medical Association, London.

67. Wells H.G. (1934). *The Work, Wealth and Happiness of Mankind*, Heinemann, London.

68. Goldstone L.A. (1983). *Understanding Medical Statistics*, William Heinemann Medical Books Ltd, London.

INDEX